The NHS and Contemporary Health Challenges From a Multilevel Perspective

Louise Dalingwater
Sorbonne Université, France

A volume in the Advances in Healthcare Information Systems and Administration (AHISA) Book Series

IGI Global
PUBLISHER of TIMELY KNOWLEDGE

Published in the United States of America by
IGI Global
Medical Information Science Reference (an imprint of IGI Global)
701 E. Chocolate Avenue
Hershey PA, USA 17033
Tel: 717-533-8845
Fax: 717-533-8661
E-mail: cust@igi-global.com
Web site: http://www.igi-global.com

Library of Congress Cataloging-in-Publication Data

Names: Dalingwater, Louise, author.
Title: The NHS and contemporary health challenges from a multilevel perspective / Louise Dalingwater.
Description: Hershey, PA : Medical Information Science Reference, [2020] | Includes bibliographical references and index. | Summary: "This book illustrates the complexities of governing public health services and examines contemporary health challenges facing the National Health Service from a multilevel perspective"-- Provided by publisher.
Identifiers: LCCN 2020000795 (print) | LCCN 2020000796 (ebook) | ISBN 9781799839286 (hardcover) | ISBN 9781799839293 (ebook)
Subjects: MESH: Great Britain. National Health Service. | National Health Programs | Health Policy | Delivery of Health Care | United Kingdom
Classification: LCC RA441 (print) | LCC RA441 (ebook) | NLM WA 540 FA1 | DDC 362.1--dc23
LC record available at https://lccn.loc.gov/2020000795
LC ebook record available at https://lccn.loc.gov/2020000796

This book is published in the IGI Global book series Advances in Healthcare Information Systems and Administration (AHISA) (ISSN: 2328-1243; eISSN: 2328-126X)

British Cataloguing in Publication Data
A Cataloguing in Publication record for this book is available from the British Library.

All work contributed to this book is new, previously-unpublished material.
The views expressed in this book are those of the authors, but not necessarily of the publisher.

For electronic access to this publication, please contact: eresources@igi-global.com.

Advances in Healthcare Information Systems and Administration (AHISA) Book Series

ISSN:2328-1243
EISSN:2328-126X

Editor-in-Chief: Anastasius Moumtzoglou, Hellenic Society for Quality & Safety in Healthcare and P. & A. Kyriakou Children's Hospital, Greece

MISSION

The **Advances in Healthcare Information Systems and Administration (AHISA) Book Series** aims to provide a channel for international researchers to progress the field of study on technology and its implications on healthcare and health information systems. With the growing focus on healthcare and the importance of enhancing this industry to tend to the expanding population, the book series seeks to accelerate the awareness of technological advancements of health information systems and expand awareness and implementation.

Driven by advancing technologies and their clinical applications, the emerging field of health information systems and informatics is still searching for coherent directing frameworks to advance health care and clinical practices and research. Conducting research in these areas is both promising and challenging due to a host of factors, including rapidly evolving technologies and their application complexity. At the same time, organizational issues, including technology adoption, diffusion and acceptance as well as cost benefits and cost effectiveness of advancing health information systems and informatics applications as innovative forms of investment in healthcare are gaining attention as well. **AHISA** addresses these concepts and critical issues.

COVERAGE

- Pharmaceutical and Home Healthcare Informatics
- E-Health and M-Health
- Measurements and Impact of HISA on Public and Social Policy
- Management of Emerging Health Care Technologies
- Clinical Decision Support Design, Development and Implementation
- Nursing Expert Systems
- IS in Healthcare
- Rehabilitative Technologies
- IT Applications in Physical Therapeutic Treatments
- Virtual health technologies

IGI Global is currently accepting manuscripts for publication within this series. To submit a proposal for a volume in this series, please contact our Acquisition Editors at Acquisitions@igi-global.com or visit: http://www.igi-global.com/publish/.

The Advances in Healthcare Information Systems and Administration (AHISA) Book Series (ISSN 2328-1243) is published by IGI Global, 701 E. Chocolate Avenue, Hershey, PA 17033-1240, USA, www.igi-global.com. This series is composed of titles available for purchase individually; each title is edited to be contextually exclusive from any other title within the series. For pricing and ordering information please visit http://www.igi-global.com/book-series/advances-healthcare-information-systems-administration/37156. Postmaster: Send all address changes to above address.

Titles in this Series

For a list of additional titles in this series, please visit:
https://www.igi-global.com/book-series/advances-healthcare-information-systems-administration/37156

Computational Intelligence and Soft Computing Applications in Healthcare Managemet Science
Muhammet Gul (Munzur University, Turkey) Erkan Celik (Munzur University, Turkey) Suleyman Mete (Gaziantep University, Turkey) and Faruk Serin (Munzur University, Turkey)
Medical Information Science Reference • © 2020 • 322pp • H/C (ISBN: 9781799825814) • US $295.00

Handbook of Research on Advancements of Artificial Intelligence in Healthcare Egineering
Dilip Singh Sisodia (National Institute of Technology, Raipur, India) Ram Bilas Pachori (Indian Institute of Technology, Indore, India) and Lalit Garg (University of Malta, Malta)
Medical Information Science Reference • © 2020 • 420pp • H/C (ISBN: 9781799821205) • US $385.00

Evaluating Challenges and Opportunities for Healthcare Reform
Raj Selladurai (Indiana University Northwest, USA) Charlie Hobson (Indiana University Northwest, USA) Roshini Isabell Selladurai (In His Image Family Medicine Residency, Ascension St. John Medical Center, USA) and Adam Greer (Ascension St. John Medical Center, USA)
Medical Information Science Reference • © 2020 • 287pp • H/C (ISBN: 9781799829492) • US $275.00

Managing Patients' Organizations to Improve Healthcare Emerging Research and Opportunities
Francesca Costanza (University LUMSA, Palermo, Italy)
Medical Information Science Reference • © 2020 • 173pp • H/C (ISBN: 9781799826538) • US $195.00

Handbook of Research on Optimizing Healthcare Management Techniques
Nilmini Wickramasinghe (Swinburne University of Technology, Australia & Epworth HealthCare, Australia)
Medical Information Science Reference • © 2020 • 431pp • H/C (ISBN: 9781799813712) • US $365.00

Table of Contents

Preface

This book project began a few years ago when, after undertaking extensive research on health services in Britain, I started to draw together many of the various insights gained from extensive study of the wealth of literature on public healthcare services. It has also offered the opportunity to share some empirical work on National Health Service (NHS) provision in the United Kingdom.

At the final stages of the project, after review in February 2020, a one in a lifetime global pandemic started to take its toll across the globe. In light of the Covid-19 pandemic, which is putting unprecedented pressure on public health institutions across the world, this book offers a timely insight into many of the public healthcare challenges facing our health institutions today. It applies health policy analysis to the area of health services. Health policy analysis is a multidisciplinary approach taken to study public policy in order to explain the interaction between institutions, interests and ideas in the policy process. It seems particularly relevant to use such an approach to study the NHS because it implies taking both a retrospective and prospective approach to understanding past policy failures and successes and to plan for future policy implementation.

Taking a multidisciplinary approach, the publication aims to illustrate the complexities of governing public health services. The main thesis is that the current NHS governance model is problematic because of the tensions between the various actors: political, economic, social and legal stakeholders, who are very often working to different agendas. So far, reforms to try and improve the running of the NHS through the introduction of market mechanisms or increased decentralisation have only served to exacerbate such tensions and resulted in further fragmentation of the public healthcare system. This work draws on insights from several academic disciplines including medicine, public health, economics, social sciences and humanities in order to navigate across the complex governance issues of public healthcare services, working at different scalar levels from the local to the global level.

This publication is fairly ambitious in scope, looking at the governance of public health services from many different perspectives. It raises the various challenges that clinical staff, public authorities, the general public and local, national and international players face in the provision of healthcare to uphold many of the core values inherent in health systems and notably, solidarity, community, equity and dignity. It will be of particular interest to scholars and students analysing the key questions and policies relating to health policy, health services and trade and investment in public services. These are current topics of debate because governments and health stakeholders are facing the dilemma of how to cope with financial pressures and increasing demand for health services.

Although this is not a textbook, its multidisciplinary nature and the diversity of topics covered under a coherent theme could make it a useful learning tool for undergraduate, but especially graduate students, working in a broad range of fields, for a large variety of courses relating to health but also international politics, trade and investment: health policy and practice, health economics, international political economy, international politics and international trade and investment. More generally, it should appeal to the general public who wish to learn more about the workings of one of the biggest employers in Europe, the NHS.

Chapter 1 offers a short history of changes to governance structures since the introduction of market-based reforms in the UK. From 1979 onwards, it is clear that market governance has been central in the delivery of public health services in the UK. The move towards using private sector techniques to run public health services has been reinforced over the last few decades and New Public Management (NPM) reforms have often been more pronounced than in many other European countries. The chapter considers how public health services have been reconfigured within the changing boundaries between the state and its citizens. The government still continues to play a major role in the running of health services and decision making, even in the new configuration of public health services and the extension of informal networks, but health policy is also now formulated through a variety of different actors. This chapter will finish by presenting how healthcare is organised today in the UK, following these reforms, so that readers who are not familiar with the public health system in the UK can gain an understanding of how the institutions which make up the NHS work.

Chapter 2 focuses on financial governance in the NHS. Faced with significant difficulties to meet financial costs owing to increased demand for healthcare, NHS organisations are looking to maintain tight financial control and reduce expenditure where possible. Significant price hikes in essential medicines can also raise challenges to the supply of necessary drugs for the population. The NHS continues to supply healthcare free at the point of use and any attempts to introduce charges remain unpopular. There have been a number of ways in which providers endeavour to reduce costs: rationalisation (reduction of services or certain costly drugs) or through increasing the role of private providers in healthcare provision. This chapter thus reviews the funding challenges the NHS is currently facing and how financial governance is evolving to meet those challenges.

Chapter 3 looks at the key workers in the NHS. Professional practitioners, in particular doctors and nurses, have a key role to play in the running of the NHS, but there are many challenges in managing staff and especially ensuring high retention levels. This chapter begins by explaining the power relations within the NHS and among some of the key actors. It then highlights some of the workforce challenges including those posed by the loss of EU staff following the UK's decision to leave the EU. In particular, it explains why it has become increasingly difficult in recent years to retain staff in the NHS. It then discusses some of the measures to stem the haemorrhaging of staff.

Chapter 4 considers the challenges to providing a person and public inclusive approach within the NHS. Person and public involvement (PPI) in healthcare provision has become an essential part of the governance framework of the NHS today. Patient safety, quality and responsiveness of care is one of the main priorities of national healthcare providers. Yet in practice, there are significant limitations to the introduction of a true patient- or person-centred approach which will be described in this chapter. Two case studies have been included to illustrate the challenges to implementing a true person-centred approach in the NHS. The first relates to the Mid-Staffordshire hospital trust where hundreds of patients died as a result of sub-standard levels of care. The second focuses on a family's struggle to access a joined-up package of care for a Parkinson's disease sufferer in a primary care setting.

Chapter 5 deals with the place-based challenge. When considering the provision of healthcare services, it is necessary to examine action at a local level and problems that local health service providers must face. This is essentially because it is within individual communities and neighbourhoods that most public healthcare interventions take place. Local intervention is also important in order to co-ordinate a more even pattern of healthcare provision across the regions. There are significant disparities between regions and inter-regions of the UK. Recent cuts to public services, welfare benefits and public employment have severely affected those regions. This chapter will thus explore health inequalities and inequities of supply across the devolved administrations, regions and sub-regions. It will then review policy to address health inequalities and consider to what extent the current public health service governance framework, and especially health service provision at the local level, can mitigate disparities in health outcomes.

Chapter 6 extends the analysis of chapter 5 to look more specifically at how localities are working towards integrated models of care. Delivering high quality health and social care is considered to be one of the key governance challenges in the UK. People are living longer and chronic diseases are more prevalent, which puts ever more pressure on health and social services to deliver. In order to better co-ordinate these services and deal with increased demand and funding pressures, authorities at both national and local levels are moving towards integrated care services. However, the integration of these services is plagued with difficulties. This chapter will explore the complexities of joining-up health and social care. It includes a case study of Continuing Healthcare (CHC), which is a package of care provided by the NHS and which involves a number of providers across the health and social care sectors. While much of the chapter focuses on health and social care challenges in England, it will finish with analysis of Scotland's progress towards integrated services.

Chapter 7 presents the specific challenges of the move towards a fully digitalised NHS. The benefits of a fully digitalised public healthcare system are significant. Digital health is an essential tool in order to improve efficiency, provide co-ordinated care and make real health improvements. However, the NHS has yet to provide a fully digitalised system to patients and providers despite technological advances in recent years. This chapter will describe the progress which has already been made in providing remote health services within the NHS. It will also explore problems arising from digitalising health services and the management of health both within the institution and through more informal networks beyond the NHS.

Chapter 8 \ differs somewhat in its approach to governance issues compared with the previous chapters as it goes beyond the national framework. In essence, the national and sub-national issues at stake do not quite capture the full picture when considering the future challenges of the provision of public healthcare services in the UK. This chapter looks at healthcare service exchanges across borders. Indeed, there has been a significant expansion of services trade, and in particular health services, which have grown not only thanks to a number of institutional frameworks but also to the support of the British government and health stakeholders. However, there are also a number of risks involved in the international exchange of health services which can have a significant impact on public healthcare systems.

In sum, across eight chapters, this book offers a kaleidoscope of many of the governance challenges facing the NHS in the UK today.

Acknowledgment

I would like to acknowledge the help and support of my family, friends and colleagues and, in particular, Martine Azuelos, Susan Finding, Jacques-Henri Coste, Jean-Baptiste Velut, Vanessa Boullet and Jacqueline Dalingwater. I would also like to thank the anonymous peer reviewers for the very helpful comments to improve the original manuscript and IGI Global Publishers for their timely support and advice.

Introduction

Most British people have a special place in their hearts for the National Health Service (NHS), even if they have not had the misfortune of experiencing the trauma of bypass or cardiovascular surgery. Far from the image of a bureaucratic monster too big to control, they believe that the essential ingredients of the public good are inherent in the NHS, even in England, the one nation of the United Kingdom that has perhaps experienced the greatest transformation in public healthcare provision since the regional separation of health management in the 1990s.

While neoliberal policy has eroded much of the British social contract[1] and resulted in state retrenchment for many public services such as education, transport and the like, the essential foundations of the social contract would appear to have been upheld in the public health domain since the foundation of the NHS in 1948. Perhaps this is because there will always be an essential "veil of ignorance"[2] about one's future health and there has never been any doubt that the creation of the NHS has, in the words of its creator, Aneurin Bevan, "lifted the shadow of fear from the homes of millions"[3].

Countries differ in the way that healthcare systems work. There are indeed a wide variety of healthcare systems functioning across the world. However, in terms of financial types, two main distinctions can be made: Bismarkian health systems (financed through social insurance contributions), and Beveridge health systems (financed through National Insurance (NI) contributions and taxation) (Rothgang, 2009). The way in which the healthcare system is regulated may also lead to different classifications, for example 'state-led', 'corporatist-governed' and 'market-driven systems' (Giaimo & Manow, 1999). Moran also identifies 'the supply state', 'the corporatist state' and 'the insecure command and control state' (Moran, 2000). More generally, it is also possible to distinguish between three types of health systems: national health services, social insurance systems and private healthcare systems.

Britain pioneered the Beveridge system by establishing the NHS in 1948. Britain has a national health service system and uses a so-called 'single-payer' model – whereby healthcare is free at the point of use, paid for out of taxation, and health workers are employees of the government. Britain, like most OECD countries, has universal or near universal coverage of healthcare for a number of key and costly health services: consultations with doctors and specialists, tests and examinations and surgical and therapeutic procedures. Public expenditure covers 80% of all healthcare costs here (OECD, 2015). However, dental care and pharmaceutical drugs are often excluded from coverage (OECD, 2015). There is a universal notion to this kind of support because the citizen has health cover and not just the worker. Tax-funded systems tend to guarantee greater equal and universal access to health for its citizens. The majority of the British working population thus pays into the public health service system and all receive treatment free at the point of use. Nevertheless, around 10% of the population is covered by some form of supplementary private health insurance (Papanicolas, Mossialos, Abel-Smith, Gundersen, & Woskie, 2019).

The NHS was founded on two pieces of legislation dating back to 1948. The NHS Act created the National Health Service and another important act, the National Assistance Act, which commissioned local authorities to provide welfare for the disabled, sick and aged (social care). It put an end to the Poor Laws[4]. Social care however has since been provided on a needs and means-tested basis. Much of social care is thus paid for privately. The 1948 Act has since been replaced by the National Health Service Act 1977, the National Health Service Act 2006 and finally the Health and Social Care Act of 2012.

However, the notion of health as a public good[5], which is enshrined in the founding legislation of the NHS, began to be undermined towards the end of the 1960s. This publication will focus on the period when such a transformation started to take place and notably from 1979 when the New Right Conservative government arrived in power. Faced with fiscal crisis and economic stagnation, academics and policymakers alike began to criticise the Keynesian post-war framework that had been set up. The rationale underlying the public provision and financing of healthcare was called into question because it became all the more difficult for governments to fund the rising costs of healthcare. Progress in medical treatments and healthcare techniques led to increased life expectancy, which meant that an ageing population put ever more pressure on the health system to maintain its population in good health. Such financial pressures and economic realities paved the way for a new political paradigm. Texts by post-war theorists such as Friedrich Hayek argued that the spontaneous order of the market was superior to planned societies with big government. Public choice theorists, Buchanan (1967, 1968) and Tullock (1962) among others, claimed that individuals and groups all had a vested interest in supporting the growth of public services, which lead to over-production and waste. Bacon & Eltis (1976) suggested that there had been a crowding out of the private sector because of the post-war expansion of the public sector, which was detrimental to the economy. Such ideas were exposed and debated at the Mont Pelerin Society where academics and politicians talked about the benefits of free-enterprise policies over Keynesian state involvement. They were then taken up by influential politicians of the New Right in the 1970s, which led to the development of a New Public Management (NPM) approach when Margaret Thatcher came to power in 1979. One of the areas in which reforms were introduced as a result of the influence of these pro-market neoliberal thinkers was in the health domain. Since the 1980s, the British health system has experienced significant reforms, with a number of attempts to introduce market mechanisms into the NHS.

A vast literature has emerged on the progressive privatisation of the NHS as a result of the overhaul of public services. In *NHS Plc*. Allyson Pollock, Professor of Public Health Research and Policy, accuses successive governments of "corroding the fabrics of the NHS at every level" and turning the NHS into a state company for profit (a plc.) (Pollock 2004, p.1). Some works have gone further and condemned successive governments for dismantling and privatising the NHS: such as White's *Who Really Runs Britain?: The Private Companies Taking Control of Benefits, Prisons, Asylum, Deportation, Security, Social Care and the NHS* (2017), or the publication by Davis, Lister and Wrigley *NHS for Sale: Myths, Lies & Deception* (2005), or Player and Leys *The Plot Against the NHS* (2011). However, in some areas, the government is currently making a U-turn on contracting out services to the private sector, for example by announcing in the 2018 autumn budget statement that there would be no future negotiations of Private Finance Initiatives (PFIs). Nevertheless, the reconfiguration of the NHS by successive governments and the changing nature of demand for healthcare have meant that public health services are no longer considered from a purely public good perspective. Financial pressures, the redefinition of health and social care and globalisation have transformed public healthcare. However, it would appear that the process of change is perhaps more complex than it first appears. The transformations have not led to the same degree of marketisation in public healthcare as in other public services. To what extent the fabric of the NHS has been corroded is thus debatable. Despite successive reform bills, no government or entity has completely unpicked the social contract upheld by the original legislation which guarantees that public health services remain free at the point of use. This is in contrast to the high out-of-pocket costs in higher education, transport and other public services.

Yet, the degree of privatisation or corrosion of the NHS foundations is not the central theme of this publication. While supporting to some extent the observations on the corrosive nature of recent reforms of the NHS and showing how the British health system is indeed increasingly subject to market mechanisms, this publication takes a different approach. Its main focus is the complexity of governance issues and the contentious interaction of actors across the acute, primary and secondary care settings[6] in the delivery of public healthcare. Many publications choose to separate such actors or clearly distinguish the private from the public. This publication wishes to show the complex merging of the public and the market in public healthcare provision. It shows how tensions arise between governors (the state, legislators, commissioners and provider networks) and the governed (the British population) on what healthcare should be provided and at what cost.

Governance of the health sector in Britain is thus the central theme of this publication. One way of bringing together the different trends in healthcare delivery at all spatial levels is through an analysis of governance frameworks at these various levels. Governance might be defined as the framework through which political, economic, social and administrative authority is exercised at local, national and international levels (Osborne, 2010).

While the nature and scope of governance is much debated in the literature, four main meanings for the term governance can be identified in specific contexts (Klijn & Koppenjan, 2014). The first is good governance, or what is sometimes referred to as corporate governance, which underlines the principles of a properly functioning public administration which should include fair treatment of citizens and an organisation that adheres to the basic principles of law. Governance as New Public Management (NPM), which has also sometimes been referred to as market governance (Hood, 1991; Osborne & Gaebler 1992) is the second common interpretation of governance. According to this definition, the role of governments is described as that of steering public service delivery rather than rowing (Osborne & Gaebler, 1992). While governments are still responsible for setting the goals and formulating policies, the delivery of services is left to separate public agencies held accountable through the setting of performance indicators, targets and by using other market mechanisms such as contracts, competition and benchmarks. However, it has often been argued that NPM is not really related to governance at all. NPM, which involves steering at a distance with market mechanisms to improve, but also to reduce the size of bureaucracy, is in some ways an opposing paradigm to governance because it still emphasises the role of central steering. NPM can be considered to actually reinforce vertical relations, whereas governance tends to emphasise horizontal relationships (Klijn & Koppenjan, 2015).

The third strand of governance which is often underlined in the literature, and is very relevant in the current context when we look beyond the national level, is multilevel governance. Networks at both local and international levels are seen to be vital for the delivery of public services. Specific types of networks with public actors at various governmental levels have significant roles to play (Agranoff & McGuire, 2003; Klijn & Koppenjan, 2015). It is only when we move from the national to the local and supranational levels that governance of health services and health service delivery are most apparent. The notions of state and society have also become increasingly blurred because de facto networks involving public and private actors have taken over service delivery. It contradicts the dominant Weberian perspective that sees governing to be based on a tight cluster of connected institutions. The NHS at the local level has been driven by the move from Weberian administration to the NPM-managerial approach to service delivery, which aims at being patient or customer-friendly but also functioning as a service enterprise, and it is clear that the two are sometimes at odds with each other (Schedler & Proeller, 2000; Kuhlmann & Bouckaert, 2016). The arm's-length governance approach in health services has been rolled out through a succession of exchanges but also challenges between the governors (those who provide the service) and the governed (the population). As Kooiman (2003) underlines, beyond the day to day management of health services, there is a process of setting rules to favour specific institutional arrangements. Bevir (2013) shows how governance is all about political contestation and rests on competitive webs of belief, which will become apparent in this publication, particularly when we look at the challenges of managing the division between health and social care, but also in the final chapter which describes the expansion of health services at an international level. Finally, much emphasis is put on network governance: the complex interaction of networks of public, private and societal actors which may be individuals, groups and/or organisations. Network governance of course is enhanced with the increasing move towards digitalised health services.

All these definitions are relevant to our analysis of the NHS in the UK and help us understand the process of governing within this giant organisation.

Analysis of governance within the NHS also reveals the role and limits of governmental power. However, it should be noted that some of the analysis in subsequent chapters, which describe processes of service delivery, is not necessarily about governance at all. In some aspects of healthcare delivery, we are still confronted with classical hierarchical bureaucracies. The following chapters will thus describe both governance processes and these traditional hierarchical bureaucracies in the delivery of public healthcare services.

The relationship between the governors (service providers, the government) versus the governed (some front line staff of the NHS and patients) which will be described in this publication contradicts much of rational choice theory which posits that humans are goal directed and that they understand their environment. It assumes that the decision makers (the governors) have complete information. However, the literature on governance and governance networks discounts this and underlines three types of complexities in governance processes. The first is substantive complexity in that, contrary to neoclassical belief, governance actors (stakeholders in the delivery of health services) are not fully informed, knowledge is uncertain and contested on the nature of the problem and the desirable solutions. The second complexity is strategic. There is an unpredictability of strategies that the various actors of service delivery will use, depending on capacity and what instruments are available. Finally, institutional complexity depends on the interaction of various actors, with different rules applying (Klijn & Koppenjan, 2015). Due to such complexities, the governors or health providers often terminate their search for information before they come to the optimal option, which may lead to governance failure. Cognitive, cultural and institutional theories also come into play because the decision makers are also using cultural biases to take action and choose who to blame when governance processes break down. Governors and governance networks may fail in their endeavours to service the population for a number of reasons: high transaction costs of the partnerships, discrepancy between the temporal and spatial horizons of the actors and lack of capacity to steer the system. Lack of accountability is also a key aspect when considering service delivery and inefficiencies in the governance of systems (Sorensen & Torfing, 2007).

This publication thus begins by describing how governance patterns have evolved since the late 1970s. It focuses on the increasing financial pressures. It considers the central actors of the healthcare system: the front-line workers and the patients. It then moves on to look at the specific nature of governance at different multiscalar levels. The transformation of governance and indeed government involvement in managing and steering the NHS is evident when we go beyond the national framework to look at how the NHS has a very distinct role in the localities. It is something that may have been overlooked in previous publications on the NHS. The move towards the digitalisation of healthcare further reinforces the multiscalar level of health service provision. This publication also shows how the internationalisation of public health systems, while perhaps not an immediate concern, may have serious consequences for the future provision of public healthcare in Britain. It thus takes stock of many new developments in the NHS.

A number of publications on the NHS have tended to see the institution as one whole, with clear divisions into acute care, primary care, etc. However, this monograph chooses not to describe the hospital sector and the primary setting separately for the very reason that the dividing line and relations between the two are becoming increasingly blurred. The same is true for the division between health and social care, mental and physical health. This publication will thus not treat the NHS as one whole. It contends that there is not one national health service but a network of health services, sometimes working together but very often fragmented and working according to different agendas.

This current volume will thus bring together research perspectives in an area that particularly lends itself to a multidisciplinary approach. While medicine and public health tend to dominate the area of public health research, the issues covered in this monograph, relating to governance, the geography of healthcare provision, globalisation and internationalisation of public healthcare services, imply that there is an overlap into other disciplines. This publication thus draws on insights from several academic disciplines including medicine, public health, economics, social sciences and humanities in order to navigate across the complex governance issues of public health services, working at different scalar levels from the local to the global level.

The present publication thus aims to illustrate the complexities of governing public health services which are part of the NHS. The main thesis is that the current NHS governance model is problematic because of the tensions between the various governors: political, economic, social and legal stakeholders, who are very often working to different agendas. This is in part related to the fragmented nature of governance network processes. Governance network processes are complex because of the different nature of agendas and strategies of actors involved in health, but increasingly because of the link between social and healthcare delivery. Faced with budget constraints, strategic games are played by many actors. There is also the other issue that healthcare providers are often operating in different arenas. This makes service delivery complex (Heclo & Wildavsky, 1974; Kingdon, 2011). Recent initiatives to provide a joined-up or integrated approach are intended to solve this dilemma, but the extent of joined-up governance processes in the NHS is rather uneven. So far, reforms to try to improve the running of the NHS through the introduction of market mechanisms or increased decentralisation have only served to exacerbate such tensions and resulted in further fragmentation of the public healthcare system. Across the various chapters, the significant limits of the current governance model should become clear thanks to the examination of public healthcare provision through a multiscalar lens, which is an innovative approach.

This publication is therefore fairly ambitious in scope, looking at the governance of public healthcare services from many different perspectives. It raises the various challenges that clinical staff, public authorities, the general public and local, national and international players face in the provision of healthcare to uphold many of the core values inherent in health systems that Brown (2003) identified as solidarity, community, equity and dignity.

REFERENCES

Agranoff, R., & McGuire, M. (2003). *Collaborative public management: New strategies for local governments*. Georgetown University Press.

Bacon, R., & Eltis, W. (1976). *Britain's economic problem: Too few producers*. Macmillan.

Bevir, M. (2013). *A theory of governance*. University of California Press.

Brown, L. (2003). Comparing health systems in four countries: Lessons for the United States. *American Journal of Public Health*, *93*(1), 52–56. doi:10.2105/AJPH.93.1.52 PMID:12511384

Buchanan, J. M. (1967). *Public finance in democratic process: Fiscal institutions and individual choice*. University of North Carolina Press.

Buchanan, J. M. (1968). The demand and supply of public goods. Indianipolis: Liberty Fund Inc.

Buchanan, J. M., & Tullock, G. (1962). *The calculus of consent*. Liberty Fund. doi:10.3998/mpub.7687

Davis, J., Lister, J., & Wrigley, D. (2015). *NHS for sale: Myths, lies & deception*. Merlin Press.

Giaimo, S., & Manow, P. (1999). Adapting the welfare state - the case of healthcare reform in Britain, Germany, and the United States. *Comparative Political Studies, 32*(8), 967–1000. doi:10.1177/0010414099032008003

Heclo, H., & Wildavsky, A. (1974). *The private government of public money: Community and policy inside British politics*. Macmillan.

Hood, C. (1991). A Public Management for all Seasons. *Public Administration, 69*(2), 3–19. doi:10.1111/j.1467-9299.1991.tb00779.x

Institute of Medicine (IOM). (2003). *The future of the public's health in the 21st Century*. National Academies Press.

Kingdon, J. (2011). *Agendas, alternatives and public policies*. Longman.

Klijn, E. H., & Koppenjan, J. (2014). Complexity in governance network theory. *Complexity. Governance & Networks, 1*(1), 61–70.

Kooiman, J. (2003). *Governing as governance*. Sage.

Kuhlmann, S., & Bouckaert, G. (Eds.). (2016). *Local public sector reforms in times of crisis national trajectories and international comparisons*. Palgrave Macmillan. doi:10.1057/978-1-137-52548-2

Moran, M. (2000). Understanding the welfare state: The case of health care. *British Journal of Politics and International Relations, 2*(2), 135–160. doi:10.1111/1467-856X.00031

OECD. (2015). *Health at a glance*. OECD.

Osborne, D., & Gaebler, T. (1992). *Reinventing government: How the entrepreneurial spirit is transforming the public sector*. Addison-Wesley Publishing Company.

Osborne, S. P. (Ed.). (2010). *The new public governance? Emerging perspectives on the theory and practice of public governance*. Routledge. doi:10.4324/9780203861684

Papanicolas, I., Mossialos, E., Abel-Smith, B., Gundersen, A., & Woskie, L. (2019). Performance of UK National Health Service compared with other high income countries: Observational study. *BMJ (Clinical Research Ed.), 367*, l6326. doi:10.1136/bmj.l6326 PMID:31776110

Player, S., & Leys, C. (2011). *The plot against the NHS*. The Merlin Press.

Pollock, A. M. (2004). *NHS plc: The privatisation of our healthcare*. Verso.

Rawls, J. (1971). *A theory of justice*. HUP.

Rothgang, H. (2009). Converging governance in healthcare systems? In I. Dingeldey & H. Rothgang (Eds.), *Governance of welfare state reform. A cross national and cross sectoral comparison of policy and politics* (pp. 18–39). Edward Elgar.

Rousseau, J. J. (2012). Du contrat social, ou principes du droit politique. *Collection complète des oeuvres*. Retrieved April 16, 2020, from http://www.rousseauonline.ch/Text/du-contrat-social-ou-principes-du-droit-politique.php

Schedler, K., & Proeller, I. (2000). *New Public Management*. Paul Haupt.

Sørensen, E., & Torfing, J. (Eds.). (2007). *Theories of democratic network governance*. Palgrave Macmillan. doi:10.1057/9780230625006

White, A. (2017). *Who really runs Britain? The private companies taking control of benefits, prisons, asylum, deportation, security, social care and the NHS*. One World Publications.

ENDNOTES

1 Term which originates from Jean-Jacques Rousseau's *Du contrat social ou Principes du droit politique* and implies the legitimacy of the authority of the state over the individual. The latter consents or surrenders his or her freedom for protection of their remaining rights.

2 Philosopher John Rawls (1971) suggested that if we were blinded by a veil of ignorance and did not know our personal circumstances, we would opt for a social contract in order to protect ourselves from the unknown. This can most certainly be applied to the area of health.

3 Aneurin Bevan archives.

4 Under the Poor Laws in England, which were in place from the 16th century onwards, each parish had to look after its own poor by providing monetary relief to those who were unable to work.

5 A public good can be described as a service or good whose consumption is not dictated by the individual consumer but by society as a whole, and financed by taxation. A public good (or service) is usually one which can be consumed without reducing the amount available for others, and should not be withheld from those who cannot afford to pay for it.

6 Acute care refers to short-term, usually immediate, medical care (for example a serious illness or traumatic injury) most often provided in a hospital setting. Primary care is medical care provided by a physician, or other healthcare professional. It usually implies consulting the General Practitioner (GP): the patient's first contact with the healthcare system, who may recommend a specialist if necessary. Secondary care is specialist care.

Chapter 1
Market-Based Governance in Public Healthcare Delivery

ABSTRACT

This chapter analyses the market-based reforms introduced in the UK. From 1979 onwards, it is clear that market governance has been central in the delivery of public healthcare services in the UK. The move towards using private sector techniques to run public health services has been reinforced over the last few decades, and New Public Management (NPM) reforms have often been more pronounced than in many other European countries. The chapter considers how public health services have been reconfigured within the changing boundaries between the state and its citizens. The government still continues to play a major role in the running of health services and decision making, even in the new configuration of public health services and the extension of informal networks, but health policy is also now formulated through a variety of different actors. This chapter will finish by presenting how healthcare is organised today in the UK following these reforms.

INTRODUCTION

We are anxious to ensure that this is the start for opening up the whole of the NHS supply system so that we end up with a situation where the state is the enabler, it is the regulator, but it is not always the provider. (Tony Blair, 2003 as quoted in Pollock, 2004, p. 69)

DOI: 10.4018/978-1-7998-3928-6.ch001

As the above quote suggests, for some time now the essential day-to-day running of public services and decision making and control is no longer described as an affair of the state. Neither is it completely in the hands of the professionals that provide public services. This chapter will thus start by defining governance in relation to public health services, then consider how the National Health Service (NHS) has been reconfigured within these changing boundaries between the state and its citizens and what impact this has had on the supply of health services.

DEFINING GOVERNANCE

The term governance is said to originate from the French *gouvernance* referring to royal officers rather than the more current meaning often employed in the sense of governing or steering (Katsamunska, 2016). While 'government' and 'governance' share the same roots, they do not have the same meaning. The concept emerged traditionally as a way to describe how government steers society (Katsamunska, 2016). More recent conceptualisations have looked more closely at interaction with society, networks and the like. However, there is no common agreement on a definition for governance. In the traditional public services context, governance refers to the setting, application and enforcement of rules (Katsamunska, 2016). The concept of governance has also been extended to the company level under the framework of 'corporate governance', which looks at management practices in companies. In the 1980s, the UK was one of the first countries to apply corporate governance practices within the public sector in line with the emergence of new leadership models (Hodges, Wright, & Keaseys, 1996).

With the reconfiguration of health services in the UK, and in particular in England, the notion of governance has been used to describe the whole framework of stakeholders who are involved in decision making and the running of services in Britain. Bevir and Rhodes (2003) define governance as the changing boundaries between the British state and civil society, with informal authority and networks taking on the authority of government.

According to Offe, the reason why there is much recent discourse on governance is that state policy and hierarchical forms of imposing action have failed to solve the problems in many areas of public life (Offe, 2009). This has thus given way to policy-making through networks, market and quasi-market solutions which steer public service provision (Enroth, 2014). The introduction of market mechanisms in the 1980s led to a fragmentation of service delivery and, to make up for this, a range of inter-organisational co-ordination in the form of networks took place (Rhodes, 1997; Enroth, 2014). In the same way, the introduction of New Public Management (NPM), which Rhodes (1997) describes as a new form of governance, has received a lot of criticism for having fragmented effective public service delivery.

Thus many authors reflecting on the changing face of governance in Britain claim that public service delivery has gone through three stages: a long period of Public Administration (PA) from the late 19th century to the late 1970s/ early 1980s, a second shorter period of New Public Management (NPM) which started in the 1980s and ran through to the start of the 21st century and a new 21st century trend of New Public Governance (NPG) (Osborne, 2009). However, as Osborne (2009) quite rightly underlines, this is a rather simplistic view of governance processes in the UK. This chapter focuses on the changes in the latter period with the introduction of NPM. It makes it clear that the move from NPM to NPG has not been a smooth transition and that there has been a co-existence and a continuation of NPM into the 21st century. Neither NPM nor NPG fully capture the governance processes. This chapter and subsequent ones will thus attempt to portray public policy implementation not as a dichotomy of administration versus management, but as a complex combination of the two.

In the context of public healthcare delivery, public governance can be broken down into five distinct strands. First, socio-political governance which demonstrates over-arching institutional relationships at the heart of society, which are essential in health systems. Government is no longer considered the only actor but also brings into play a number of societal actors, both health professionals and administrators, who legitimise state policy in the health field and make a real impact in the area of healthcare supply. Second, public policy governance which shows how policy elites and networks actually govern the public policy process. These are the institutions that monitor and control the health professionals to exert central control. Third, administrative governance which shows how public administration has changed and been repositioned in light of current and future complexities. Fourth, contract governance which relates to how NPM is enacted and functions: that is, the governance of contractual relationships to deliver public services and other strands of NPM. Finally, network governance is the fifth distinct strand which relates to the development of self-organising inter-organisational networks, which work with or without government to provide public services. Reforms that have been pushed through in this area have led to what has been described as "a governing out of the centre" (Osborne, 2009) and an empowerment of a variety of actors whether it be senior public servants, lower-echelon public employees or members of civil society.

There has also emerged a degree of meta-governance, that is the recognition for the need for some delegation and devolution but greater central direction, which is clear in the case of reforms under New Labour. The reforms in terms of governance have enabled greater autonomy for certain actors within the public sector, notably managers, but have also created managerial problems, which will be evident in this chapter and subsequent ones. This interactive governance system is constantly changing to keep up with inside and outside changes and challenges which affect the governors (those managing the system) and the governed (front-line staff, patients, families, etc.). This section will consider the market as a governance institution. Historically and notably since the 1970s, new forms of governance have emerged with a shift in the roles and responsibilities of bureaucracies and an increasing involvement of private institutions and agencies, partly in response to ever increasing concerns over budget constraints in the public sector, greater health demands from the population and demands for better quality services. Since governments, businesses and civil society are not able to deal with these issues on their own, they involve governance networks of relations (Marin & Mayntz, 1991; Marsh & Rhodes, 1992).

Yet the government still continues to play a major role in the running of health services and decision making, even in the new configuration of public health services and the extension of informal networks. As Ham (2009) argues, the Department of Health, which is responsible for strategic leadership and funding for both health and social care in England, is much more than a monolith. Health policy is formulated through a variety of professions, divisions and groups. However, as Rhodes claims, to some extent inter-governmental networks, a mix of governmental and societal actors, have taken the place of the government, leaving no central steer (Rhodes, 1997; Enroth, 2014). Policy co-ordination led by the Department of Health has evolved according to power struggles between different interests. The struggle in the 1980s and 1990s was seen to be between those responsible for formulating policy and those implementing policy. The NHS Executive was then integrated into the Department of Health with a significant strengthening of managerial powers. Since the 1990s, the number of stakeholders in health delivery has increased and a more complex relationship has developed as we will see in this chapter and, indeed, throughout the publication.

Beyond the strong executive influence over health policy, pressure groups may also shape the governance process, although producer groups tend to be more influential than consumer groups. Parliament, mass media, royal commissions, industrial and commercial representatives, academics and researchers may also influence policy making (Ham, 2009). It is important thus to understand the relationships between the various stakeholders who manage the NHS. Whether it be through interaction or negotiation, the Department of Health, NHS bodies and its arm's length organisations and pressure groups depend upon each other to enable health services to be provided to the population (Ham, 2009). In order to understand why new reforms and market mechanisms were introduced in the NHS from the late 1970s onwards, the general economic context which brought about such changes to public institutions will first be described.

CRISIS AND THE PATH TO REFORM

Financial Crisis and the Pressure to Reduce Expenditure

The economic and fiscal crisis which reached its zenith in the 1970s and the policy responses of the 1980s are very significant in explaining why a wholescale reform was then implemented in the NHS from the 1980s onwards. Between 1964 and 1976, Britain faced a continuing sterling crisis. The country was still suffering from the aftermath of the Second World War and its heavy debts, which were compounded by the exchange rates imposed by the Bretton Woods system. Moreover, with the collapse of the Empire, private overseas holdings of sterling currency declined (Roberts, 2016). The series of energy crises between 1967 and 1979, but especially the oil shock crisis of 1973 and the embargo imposed by Arab oil producers, severely affected the global economy and led to a stock market crash, stagflation, a combination of sky high inflation and low growth and high unemployment. In order to maintain living standards, trade unions continued to fight for higher wages. This exacerbated the inflation problem which rose above 20% in the late 1970s in Britain (Nelson & Nikolov, 2001).

In 1976, faced with crisis and convinced that the pound was over-valued, a large-scale selling of sterling took place and its value slid against the dollar. Its decline was such that the US Treasury Secretary agreed to grant a loan of $5.3 billion to support the pound, but demanded repayment in December 1976. The pressure on the pound continued and the British government was thus forced to apply to the International Monetary Fund (IMF) for a loan of

$3.9 billion in September 1976. However, such a significant loan came with a number of conditions attached, notably that Britain must reduce public expenditure and the budget deficit (Roberts, 2016). The pressure to reduce public expenditure was therefore significant.

One of the areas in which costs had continued to rise was in the area of health. The centrally funded system which relied more heavily on taxation and public expenditure than other health systems in Europe meant that the system was more sensitive to a decline in public expenditure than in other areas. On the inception of the NHS, it was assumed that the cost would be borne by local rather than national taxation, which implies that its creators had significantly underestimated the true cost of funding a universal health service. It was also impossible to imagine how costs would rise. Since the creation of the NHS in Britain, there had been significant social, demographic and technological changes. Longer life expectancy and changing patterns of diseases had meant higher demands on health services and higher costs.

The NHS and Funding Crises Before the 1980s Reforms

While significant reduction of public expenditure was called for in the 1970s, pressures to reduce expenditure and reform predate this period. Under Churchill's 1951 administration, it became clear that the financial projections for the NHS had clearly underestimated the costs and demands on public health services (Cutler, 2003; Klein, 2006; Gorsky, 2008). However, while capital investment was lower than the 1930s, acute hospital sector funding continued to rise (Gorsky, 2008). In the 1960s, the NHS benefited from a significant rise in expenditure until 1972. In the early 1970s, public health had made outstanding progress, mainly thanks to advances in medical science. The NHS was seen to be performing well and able to offer transplants for the first time, intensive care units were becoming widely available, the first Computerised Axial Tomography (CAT) scan, which enabled cross-sectional X-rays of the human body, was provided by the NHS. The General Practitioner (GP) charter was introduced in order to improve and expand the provision of primary care in the UK. A number of health centres were subsequently opened across the country. The first computers were introduced into NHS hospitals and overall it was considered that people were getting better standards of care.

However, owing to rising costs, there was a debate about the sustainability of the NHS and the necessity to bring about reforms to ensure the future provision of public health services to the nation (BBC, 2002). This was exacerbated by the fiscal and economic crisis. Towards the mid-1970s, tensions started to rise with cuts to services as governments were forced to rein in spending following the restrictions imposed by the IMF loan. The next section will describe in more detail the system in place prior to the 1980s and how this system was gradually dismantled.

THE RECONFIGURATION OF PUBLIC HEALTH SERVICES IN BRITAIN

Traditional Public Administration (PA) and the NHS

Upon its creation, services in the NHS were divided into hospital and specialist services, family practitioner services (GP, pharmaceutical services, dentist and ophthalmic services) and community services (maternity, child welfare, midwifery, health visiting, home nursing, domestic help, prevention, care, aftercare, ambulances, mental health) (Abel-Smith, 1978; Grimmeisen & Frisina, 2010). Traditional PA in the NHS up until the 1980s was characterised by a system split between political bureaucracy and the professions. It was a decentralised system in which the Department of Health maintained a loose control to ensure adequate resources, quality and quantity of service provision.

When the conservatives were elected into government in 1979, there were 14 Regional Health Authorities, 90 Area Health Authorities and 192 District Health Authorities (DHAs). The Area Health Authorities were divided according to local authority boundaries whereas DHAs covered the catchment areas in which district general hospitals were located. DHAs were allocated funds from the Department of Health according to a capitation formula and hospitals negotiated an operating budget. The Resource Allocation Working Group, set up in 1975, was responsible for allocating resources for secondary care according to need. The system was supposedly characterised by a 'command and control' or top-down system with the district management team responsible for managing and imposing their will on employees to ensure the high performance of hospitals. However, in practice, the medical profession was organised in clans who controlled the delivery of health services and imposed their own mode of governance. Outwardly, the hospital reflected the model of the professional bureaucracy. Doctors were thought and assumed to act in the best interest of their patients and therefore they could enjoy autonomy and self-regulation.

However, in the 1970s, this mode of governance came increasingly under attack. Towards the end of the 1970s, despite significant medical progress, measures of performance showed that healthcare delivery was suffering from these inefficiencies. Excessive waiting times for treatment and variable quality of care meant that the public became increasingly critical of the ability of doctors and professionals to manage healthcare (Lapsley, 1994; Le Grand, 2003).

New Public Management (NPM)

NPM developed as a reaction to post-war PA principles. Towards the end of the 1960s, in light of the fiscal crisis and economic stagnation, academics began to call into question the post-war framework that had been set up. Public choice theorists[1] claimed that clinicians were acting through self-interest rather than for the public good. Indeed, Buchanan and Tullock (1962) argued that interest groups, given too much power, were capable of determining the patterns of public expenditure. In order to remove such distortions, public choice theorists promoted free-market policies and limited state involvement. Hayek (1944), whose work became popular in the 1970s when he won the Nobel Memorial Prize in Economics, underlined the dangers of the growth of the public sector at the expense of the private sector. He claimed that individuals and groups all had a vested interest in supporting the growth of public services, which led to over-production and waste. According to the 'crowding-out theory', espoused by Bacon and Eltis (1976), public sector expansion was detrimental to the economy. Indeed, the authors claimed that when greater resources were allocated to public spending, private sector investment was undermined. This led to the creation of an unproductive sector at the expense of a productive one. Such ideas were exposed and debated at the Mont Pelerin Society, where academics and politicians talked about the benefits of free-enterprise policies over Keynesian state involvement. These ideas were then taken on board by influential politicians of the New Right in the 1970s and led to the development of a New Public Management approach when Margaret Thatcher came to power in 1979. The assumption of this new form of management was that private-sector managerial techniques were by and large superior to cumbersome PA principles. Such techniques if applied to public services should improve efficiency and performance. As Clarke, Leaver, and Gilbert (2015) underline, this is quite surprising when applied to the health sector given that there is no empirical evidence to suggest that the private health sector is more efficient than the public sector. NPM thus started to develop as a specific approach at the same time, and in much the same way, as neoliberalism. Some would go as far to say that the development of NPM was a way of imposing the neoliberal agenda on society through the state project NPM framework (Roberts, 2014).

Indeed, NPM developed as part of a general shift towards neoliberal attitudes and practices. Neoliberal orthodoxy posits that state intervention can create obstacles to economic and social development. NPM applies specifically to the management of public services, rather than a general orthodoxy. NPM is focused on managerial involvement to improve the quality and efficiency of public services. It emphasises the importance of public service production functions and operational issues above public service values and organisation of conventional public administration. The egalitarian ideas that were part and parcel of old administration, with a more horizontal organisation without managers and self-governance by the public service professionals, run counter to this. NPM promotes a number of techniques based on the view that the public sector can be run more efficiently if its management methods are borrowed from those that have worked well in the private sector. Nevertheless, NPM is a loose set of techniques and ideas rather than a firm paradigm. Indeed, it was only a decade after its implementation that it was identified as a framework. Christopher Hood was the first to define the nature and practice of NPM. In his article "A Public Management for all Seasons" and with specific reference to the British public sector, he listed the seven main tenets of NPM:

- Hands on professional management in the public sector
- Explicit standards and measures of performance
- Greater emphasis on output control
- Shift to disaggregation of units in the public sector
- Shift to greater competition in the public sector
- Stress on private sector styles of management practice
- Stress on greater discipline and parsimony in resource use (Hood, 1989)

Based on Hood's work, Clark (1996) grouped NPM components into three main categories:

1. Marketisation, which means introducing market competition into public services by separating the purchaser from the provider, creating 'quasi-markets' within the public sector (notably in healthcare, education, social

services and social housing), competitive tendering or outsourcing to the private sector;

2. Disaggregation, that is strengthening central strategic capacity by decoupling policy and executive functions: tighter central control over policy and frameworks, moving from concentrating on process to output in control and accountability mechanisms, and finally;
3. Incentivisation, which means creating incentives to encourage greater entrepreneurialism, more results, overall greater efficiency: performance indicators, performance-linked pay to create incentives for public sector staff to be more efficient, human resource management strategies, deprivileging professionals and public sector workers. A very reductionist form of NPM might be a three-M approach: Markets, Managers and Measurement (Clark, 1996). In practice, this was reflected in the overhaul of one of the most important public services in England: the NHS[2].

The Introduction of NPM in the NHS

NPM management techniques were introduced in the NHS after the Conservative government took office following the general election of 1979. The private sector was presented as having superior qualities to the public sector. Roy Griffiths, managing director of Sainsbury's, was brought in from the private sector to find ways in which the NHS might be governed more efficiently. His Report of 1983 was instrumental in changing the way the NHS was governed. The Griffiths report claimed that "if Florence Nightingale were carrying her lamp through the corridors of the NHS today, she would almost certainly be searching for the people in charge" (Griffiths, 1983, p.12). Griffiths thus recommended that NHS hospitals be run like private companies with strong management who would put quality and customer satisfaction first. Following the Griffiths Report of 1983, a series of political reforms were carried through to stimulate a more business-like organisation. Professional regulation and management by DHAs were replaced by Unit General Management, with managers appointed from both the public and private sectors to manage hospitals. The next step, outlined in the white paper *Working for Patients*, was to offer greater choice for patients (Department of Health, 1989). This report claimed that buying care outside the health service would relieve the NHS of its financial pressures and enable greater provision of services and thus greater choice. Public services were likened to private services with emphasis on the quality of services and value for money. DHAs were thus instructed to purchase care from private hospitals through private tendering.

As Ham (2009) underlines, the Griffith Report which led to the creation of a Health Services Supervisory Board and an NHS management board, with general managers appointed at all levels of the NHS to provide leadership, laid the foundations for the internal market created in 1991. Indeed, the managers brought in to govern the NHS were instrumental in helping push through the internal market reforms. Previously, hospitals and community services had been under the jurisdiction of DHAs and accountable to the health authorities' board (Pollock, 2004). Funds were allocated on the basis of need. No invoicing or contracting out to the private sector took place. This all changed with the implementation of the internal market. Hospitals became financially independent corporations and were responsible for making income to survive. Indeed, Compulsory Competitive Tendering, the outsourcing of non-core services such as catering and laundry, was seen to be the most effective way of involving the private sector in the provision of health services to make efficiency gains. Hospitals made money by settling contracts with NHS purchasers, who were health authorities and GPs (fund holders, given the funds to purchase hospital services on behalf of patients). This led to a restriction of services. If treatment was not considered to bring cost benefits, it was not carried out.

Indeed, the problem of granting money to the authorities and GP fund holders meant that some were allocated more funding than others to spend on patients, which exacerbated the infamous "postcode lottery", whereby the standard of healthcare and supply depended on the district in which you lived (Pollock, 2004). The hospital management team was reviewed on its performance. Clinical needs were thus less important now than efficiency criteria. Hospitals might refuse patients to meet performance targets and, at the end of the year, whole wards or theatres had to close down if the hospital overspent. In addition, GP fund holders would often retain surpluses from their budgets to invest in their practices and avoid taking on high risk and costly patients (Pollock, 2004). To meet these new rationing orders and make efficiency savings, many mergers took place.

Moreover, the NHS and Community Care Act of 1990 confirmed the gradual takeover of quasi-market forms of governance, which were part and parcel of NPM. In order to take on the role of health providers, health authorities who purchased health services had to become NHS trusts. In addition, GP fund holders were created who could purchase services directly from providers instead of going via the Health Authority. The intention was eventually that the GP fund holders would replace the commissioning carried out by the Health Authorities. The creation of NHS trusts reinforced the separation between the purchaser and provider. The trusts were self-governing, non-profit provider organisations financed by public capital. There was also emphasis on outputs and outcomes and key targets were introduced in the NHS. Thus, massification of services, cost effectiveness, customer choice, performance management and performance-related pay for health professionals became the key features of the new NHS under NPM reforms.

However, a decade after its application NPM also came under fire for its lack of a real theoretical basis, for its questionable benefits and the difficulties inherent in applying private sector techniques to the public sphere, and especially health services. Towards the end of the 1990s, it came to be seen as one-dimensional, failing to be effective in the management and governance of health services and leading to fragmentation in the delivery of public services (Lapsley, 1994; Le Grand, 2003).

Moreover, the British healthcare system was in a critical state in the 1990s. Services were unable to meet demand; people were reported to be dying on waiting lists because, despite organisational changes, there was a lack of investment in public healthcare services. According to two influential reports, written by Derek Wanless, successive governments had failed to invest in the NHS (Wanless, 2002; Wanless, 2004). The performance of the British health system was well below that of its European counterparts (OECD, 2014). The debate on whether the changes had brought efficiency gains was therefore foreclosed because of lack of investment.

Post-NPM, New Public Governance and Clinical Governance

When New Labour was elected into government in 1997 a number of problems associated with the NPM mode of governance in the NHS were identified, such as the absence of clear incentives to improve performance, the disempowerment of patients, a lack of national standards and variations in treatment. Moreover, the original intention of the internal market was to create competition between hospitals and thus make efficiency and quality gains. However, the working of the internal market was undermined by lack of investment in the NHS (Webster, 2002; Klein, 2006).

New Labour heralded a new, third way approach which removed the excesses of NPM by scrapping the internal market and performance management targets in public health. Indeed, the white paper *The New NHS: Modern, Dependable*, published in 1997, shortly after the change in government, stated the changes to be neither going back to the old bureaucratic PA system nor embracing NPM: "...no return to the old centralised command and control system of the 1970s [nor] the divisive internal market of the 1990s (...) It will be a new model for a new century" (Department of Health, 1997, p. 11). The internal market was thus replaced by commissioning and payment by results which involved a more joined-up or network-partnership approach.

Reforms were implemented in the late 1990s which altered the nature of NPM modes of governance. Devolution made it essential to bring about reforms to public management as the transfer of authority to local regulatory agencies meant that the fragmentation of service delivery, seen to be a result of NPM, had to be solved. Indeed, devolution of power implied referring the statutory granting of powers from the Parliament of the United Kingdom to the Scottish Parliament, the National Assembly for Wales, the Northern Ireland Assembly and the London Assembly and to their associated executive bodies, the Scottish Government, the Welsh Government, the Northern Ireland Executive and, in England, the Greater London Authority and combined authorities, including in the health sector. Empowering the regions also gave politicians greater incentives to ensure that central control was not completely lost and accountability and capacity were ensured. The post-NPM reforms brought in when New Labour came to power in 1997 were also made in order to improve the horizontal and vertical co-ordination of governmental organisation which had emerged out of NPM.

Indeed, from a vertical standpoint, stronger central control was also brought in to play by increasing central resources. From a horizontal point of view, post-NPM reforms focused on empowering agencies and state-owned enterprises. It also entailed bridging the gap between governance and government; that is building stronger links between the state, the private sector and civil society. New Labour discourse emphasised 'joined-up' government to mend the fragments that had been created by previous forms of governance, both PA and NPM. The aim was also to form a more cohesive structure and create more loyalty among public sector workers. Partnerships were thus encouraged between the public and private spheres as a way of integrating various areas of government action. Multilevel governance was introduced in the shape of networks and partnerships. Significant investment was also part and parcel of the post-NPM reforms. One of the most important decisions to be made under New Labour was to increase investment in the

NHS. Indeed, New Labour increased real spending between 6% and 7% a year from 2000 until 2008.

New Labour heralded the move away from NPM and referred to their new approach as Clinical Governance, that is a new quality framework, especially to respond to failures in care that had been reported: "a framework through which NHS organisations are accountable for continually improving the quality of their services and safeguarding high standards of care..." (Department of Health, 1998, p. 2). This new form of governance was initially introduced after a series of highly publicised incidents of doctors being struck off for failing to follow safety guidelines. According to Scally and Donaldson (1998), the term clinical governance was first employed after the Bristol heart scandal of 1995. It was found that babies were dying at a high rate after cardiac surgery at the Bristol Royal Infirmary. The Department of Health underlined quality issues and the need to remedy 'failure of care' (Department of Health, 1998). Clinical Governance introduced by New Labour involved streamlining and standardising processes to monitor clinical performance by developing a clear set of national standards and clear incentives to improve performance. This was achieved essentially through the introduction of clinical audit; that is review of clinical performance by setting standards and measuring those standards.

Quality management was also an important part of the clinical governance framework. Quality management was based on the thesis that while the marketplace may help efficiency, it was also necessary to redirect attention back to medical practice. The priority of New Labour thus became to set, measure and improve quality standards. The establishment of the National Institute for Health and Care Excellence (NICE) in 1999 to monitor quality management was emblematic of such new forms of governance. Since then, NICE has become an extremely influential organisation. Its role is to improve outcomes for people using the NHS and other public health and social care services in England. It produces evidence-based guidance and advice for commissioners, practitioners and managers across health and social care institutions. It develops quality standards and performance metrics to evaluate the quality of health and social care services. While doctors are not obliged to follow NICE recommendations, it proves difficult to circumvent them in practice. If, for example, practitioners or institutions choose not to give treatment recommended by NICE, they are very likely to see their decision overturned by the law courts if the patient takes legal proceedings. The National Service Framework also sets forth how care should be administered for specific diseases, disabilities and patient groups. Finally, the Commission for Health Improvement was set up to monitor and improve standards at the local level. Indeed, the poor performance of the health sector in the 1980s was in part attributed to resource misallocation. For example, people with chronic kidney failure died prematurely because of a lack of investment in dialysis, whereas investment was made to prolong life for a very short period for those with metastatic cancer at significant cost. The creation of such entities was also a response to such resource allocation dilemmas: how to estimate the cost of improving quality of life with restricted resources and how to choose the most cost-effective procedures (Aaron, Schwartz, & Cox, 2005).

New Labour also set out a reform agenda intended to deliver a more patient-centred approach to healthcare, which involved service reorganisation. Health authorities were thus to provide strategic leadership at the local level working with NHS bodies, local authorities and other partner organisations. This led to the development of Health Improvement Programmes (HImPs) which aimed at implementing national targets at the local level.

In 1999, New Labour abolished the system of fund holders because of concerns regarding inequity between patients managed by fund holders and those by non-fund holders. However, 481 Primary Care Groups (PCGs) were created in 1999 in England to take over the principles of fundholding by involving all family doctors and community nurses. Each PCG was made up of a board of four to seven GPs, one or two community or practice nurses, one social services nominee, one lay member, one health authority non-executive and the group's chief executive. While PCGs were at first advisory bodies, they could over time become Primary Care Trusts (PCTs) to commission care and provide community services (Ham, 2009). Ham views these changes as taking Conservative reforms further by extending management roles. Moreover, by giving PCGs control over resources, the latter could be transferred between acute care (hospitals) and primary care (provided in communities), thus extending the role of primary care providers in order to reduce the use of hospital services that had become over-stretched (Ham, 2009). In 2001, PCTs replaced the PCGs in all localities and at the same time the number of health authorities was reduced from 98 to 20. From 2004, PCTs became responsible for 75% of the NHS budget and were responsible for commissioning services in the localities.

Alongside PCTs, hospital trusts and care trusts were responsible for acute care. Under the Health and Social Care Act 2003, NHS hospitals and PCTs performing well were also offered the status of foundation trusts which meant that they were no longer subject to Department of Health control (Pollock, 2004; Grimmeisen & Frisina, 2010). In addition, the latter had an incentive to be as competitive as possible since they gained the right to retain and reinvest any end-of-year surpluses (Le Grand, 2002). The intention behind such reforms was to make a fundamental change from a top-down to a bottom-up approach, devolving power and decision making to patients, commissioners and clinicians (Ham, 2009). It was heralded as a joined-up approach by transferring accountability from the state to the local community in order to meet the needs of the local population. In reality, these NHS trusts had to compete and were forced to respond to market forces in order to survive. The regional offices were replaced by Strategic Health Authorities (SHAs) responsible for ensuring the performance and management of local NHS bodies. However, the proliferation of managers received criticism because it was said to have destroyed public ethos and resulted in inefficiencies (Clarke, 2007; Dillow, 2007; Dorey, 2015). Managers continued to ensure service provision of both clinical and support services.

In addition, Performance-Related Pay (PRP) was introduced to reward managers according to results. However, the OECD pointed out that there was a divergence of values between PRP and the public service ethos. Very few managers were happy with the amount they received for performance (OECD, 1997). PRP was only adopted by some institutions and abandoned by other health service providers because it created discontent among employees (Dowling & Richardson, 1997). Payment for performance also became widely used in the UK. For primary care a Quality and Outcomes Framework (QOF) was initiated to reward GP practices for hitting performance indicators. In addition, payment by results (PbR) became the new mantra for efficient delivery of health services. It implied linking the allocation of funds to hospitals in relation to the activities they undertook. Hospitals were thus paid for the activities they performed, awarded for good performance (measured by the reduction of waiting times and increased capacity) (Grimmeisen & Frisina, 2010).

As regards performance monitoring, the National Performance Assessment Framework (NPAF) was launched in June 1999 to measure and monitor key activity targets. It set out to measure performance not only in terms of efficiency, economy and effectiveness, but also quality and customer satisfaction (Kouzmin, Loffler, Klages, & Korac-Kakabadse, 1999). Targets were basically set to meet baseline requirements such as emergency pressures and financial balance, but also 'Modernisation Fund' targets such as waiting list, primary care and mental health objectives. Targets for healthcare thus became an ever important part of public health in England, although previous experience with targets had not necessarily resulted in improving efficiency in the delivery of health services.

The first official targets had been introduced in 1992, with the aim of ensuring that authorities secured good health for the population. Five key illnesses were targeted: 1. Coronary heart disease and stroke; 2. Cancers; 3. Mental illness; 4. HIV/AIDS and sexual health; and, 5. Accidents (Department of Health, 1992). However, by 1998, reports suggested that the influence of what were referred to as Health of the Nation targets were negligible in policy making. Health authorities focused more on waiting times and securing budgetary control. There was also a lack of central implication and such policy apparently failed to deal with underlying social and structural determinants of health. A large scale development of indicators however still took place in 1997 with the arrival of New Labour into power, which heralded a commitment to evidence-based policy, systematic priority setting and explicit performance targets in public services (Department of Health, 1997). In 1999, this was developed further to include indicators to evaluate access, experience, delivery, efficiency and outcomes (see Figure 1).

Figure 1. NHS Performance Assessment Framework
Source: NHS Executive (1999)

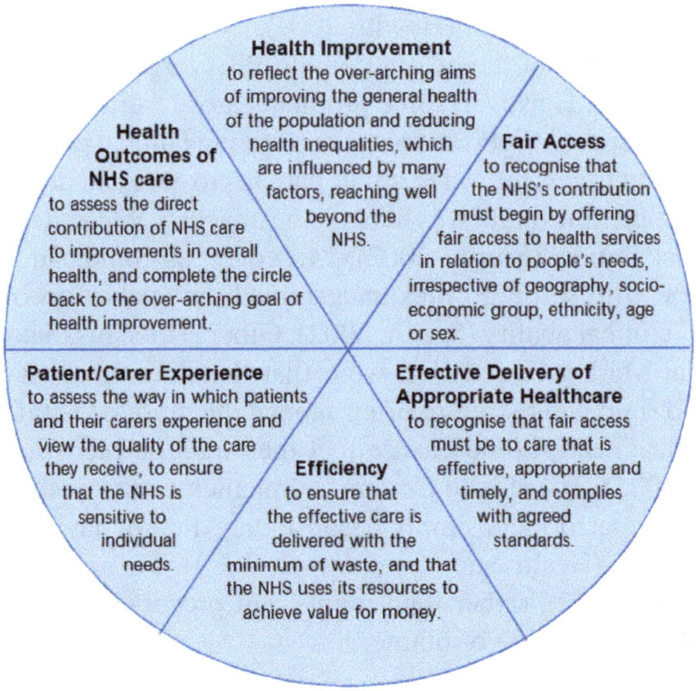

In addition, a set of Public Service Agreements (PSAs) was announced for each department to set priorities with specific targets that would be measured. PSA targets were thus set for health and social care.

Apart from more general targets to improve the health of populations (measured by life expectancy) and those with chronic diseases, specific healthcare targets were set to improve access to services, reduce waiting times and improve patient and user experience. In addition, local health authorities and NHS providers of care were also ranked annually according to their ability to perform to a composite measure of performance based on around 30 subsidiary indicators. Senior management who did not gain high performance ratings risked losing their jobs. The ratings were also used by the Department of Health to reward NHS trusts that were performing well, such as awarding them with foundation status and to sanction other trusts that were perceived to be performing poorly.

Overall, there is no clear evidence to date to suggest that quality management and clinical governance have led to greater safety or efficiency. Worse still, incidents were reported where safety was breached because of priority given to some objectives over others because of the clinical audit process. Opinions vary on the introduction of such a form of surveillance. The government defended the introduction of clinical governance, others criticised the latter for its hierarchical and elitist form of surveillance, driven by an agenda of control and risk management (Hewitt, 2007).

It would seem that in the health domain PSA targets did at first reduce NHS waiting times. However, some problems arose from these targets such as unmeasured aspects of performance, sacrificing clinical priorities in order to reduce waiting times, refusal to admit patients to accident departments if a four-hour waiting time target was likely to be unachievable and manipulation of waiting list figures (Smith, 2002). Moreover, as Smith underlines, the preoccupation with waiting times undermined the evaluation of other key indicators of clinical quality (Smith, 2002). Other criticisms that were raised by the Social Market Foundation were that there were too many targets, they were too rigid and therefore often sapped the morale of staff and it was not always clear who should ensure that the target be met (Social Market Foundation, 2005). The Health Commission lamented that some trusts were labelled as poor performers simply because they did not have the necessary performance data (Healthcare Commission, 2008). There was also greater emphasis on outcomes rather than inputs and processes and a transfer of responsibility or devolving of blame.

The involvement of the private sector was also increased under New Labour. Compulsive Competitive Tendering was replaced by Public Private Partnerships (PPPs) to outsource services to the private sector. The Prime Minister's Delivery Unit was specifically set up to manage and enforce performance management, performance indicators and PSAs. In fact, figures suggest that outsourcing health sources to private companies was actually greater under New Labour than during the previous Conservative governments. Phil Whitaker, GP and health columnist, argued that despite extra investment in health, service improvements were slow and incremental (Whitaker, 2015). Whitaker and his colleagues witnessed increasing numbers of prosperous middle class patients opting out of the state system to pay for private treatment. This led to a mantra of a new responsive and user-friendly NHS in order to keep people in public sector mode, and to avoid a crowding out of the public sector by the private sector if people were to rely more on private services than public ones. Indeed, if more people opted for private services, then this could undermine funding in the public sector. In particular, it could lead to a permanent disinvestment of public services in favour of private services. New Labour argued that the best way to be responsive was to find the most efficient way of providing high quality services, which it also believed depended on the market. From 2003 onwards, Independent Sector Treatment Centres (ISTCs) were thus opened across England. These were private healthcare organisations that provided services for NHS elective procedures and remained free of charge for NHS patients. Such contracting out did enable waiting lists to be reduced and forced existing providers to become more efficient in order to stay in the race, but contributed to a greater fragmentation of health services.

Despite the reforms that were supposed to heal fragmentation caused by NPM, it can be argued that NPM forms of governance were still prevalent. New Labour presented post-NPM reforms as a modernisation programme bringing a more collaborative approach, joined-up government and network arrangements, aimed at a less fragmented organisation of public services. These were aided by advances in new technology because networking became easier to process with the development of technology and the Internet. In reality, private sector techniques were still prioritised. Under New Labour, efficiency drives in public services were still as important as they had been during the Thatcher years. It can be argued that emphasis on responsiveness to users and giving public choice was very much in line with NPM ideas. New Labour still focused on quantifying and setting performance targets. In fact, performance targets were actually extended under New Labour.

The 2010 general elections resulted in a hung parliament. With no absolute majority, the Conservative government formed a coalition government with the Liberal Democrats. The 2008 crisis and the bank bailouts had resulted in a very significant public deficit. Both the Conservatives and Liberal Democrats pledged to cut the deficit, but not NHS funding, during the election campaign. Nevertheless, pressure was on to provide a public service which was the most efficient possible in times of fiscal retrenchment. The post-crisis coalition government thus upheld many NPM tenets. It claimed to have scrapped performance targets and developed localism[3] but there was no clear evidence that targets had disappeared. Moreover, by making cuts to local public services, local government was obliged to take on NPM-style techniques: that is find ways of making efficiency gains. In practice, it is clear to see how post-NPM modes of governance have built on NPM if we consider the reforms that have taken place more recently in the NHS (Gregory, Dixon, & Ham, 2012).

However, when the Lib-Con coalition government was formed in 2010, their discourse seemed to suggest that they would make a clear break with NPM techniques. The 2010 white paper *Equity and Excellence: Liberating the NHS* underlined how healthcare was still a public good and 'free at the point of use' (Department of Health, 2010, p.1). The coalition government also announced that national targets, a key feature of the NHS in previous governments, would be abolished. They did, however, maintain certain targets that were part of the NHS Constitution[4], such as targets for access to hospital treatment, access to cancer care and waiting times. However, the most significant reforms of the coalition government took place in 2012. The Health and Social Care Act of 2012 represented one of the most important structural changes in the history of the NHS. Embedded in this reform was the extension of choice and competition; ultimately the reinforcement of NPM ideas. The aim of this act, according to the government, was to restructure the health service in order to reduce costs, improve quality and cut bureaucracy (Dorling, 2013). Under this act, PCTs and SHAs were abolished. They were replaced by NHS England (and the equivalent in Scotland, Wales and Northern Ireland) to oversee the budget, planning, delivery and day-to-day operation of the commissioning side of the NHS in England. The PCTs were replaced by Clinical Commissioning Groups (CCGs), which were given budgets to buy care for local communities, and Health and Wellbeing Boards. The 211 CCGs thus became the main devolved purchasers of healthcare. They were henceforth in charge of health administration and made up of health professionals, general practitioners and financial administrators. A new resource allocation system was set up awarding approximately two-thirds of the total NHS budget of roughly £100 billion to CCGs to purchase general hospital, community and mental health services. The remaining third was retained by the NHS at national level, to commission primary care and specialised hospital services. However, unlike PCTs, CCGs were given the responsibility for public healthcare and not for public health (the latter was transferred to the local authorities).

The problem with the CCG model is that it puts the burden of commissioning patients' care onto GPs, who may not be qualified to carry out such tasks. The management of public health has thus been moved from the NHS to local government, although this is still overseen at a national level by a new executive government agency, Public Health England (PHE). Health and Wellbeing Boards were also created under the Health and Social Care Act of 2012 to work with the CCGs to establish health strategies for the population. Despite what would seem to be independence of different healthcare workers in this current governance framework, the House of Commons Health Committee underlined that PHE was not independent enough from government and this could mean that speaking on controversial but important public health issues may not be raised. The committee also underlined that PHE needed to both support and challenge government department policy in order to ensure that health inequalities were tackled (House of Commons Health Committee, 2015). Effective action from the centralised PHE is thus necessary even if local bodies are important.

If we look beyond the political discourse which heralds a more serious commitment to a holistic or joined-up/inter-connected approach and emphasises local forms of governance, it is possible to see that the underlying themes of NPM were still clearly at the heart of NHS reforms under the coalition government. Such tenets have been upheld by Conservative governments since 2015. The emphasis on choice that we mentioned previously is actually a key feature of NPM because the focus is also on competition to provide greater choice. The White Paper *Equity and Excellence: Liberating the NHS* states that "patients will be at the heart of everything we do. So they will have more choice and control" (Department of Health, 2010, p. 1). In addition, although the government claimed they would scrap performance targets, there is no real evidence of this in practice. Indeed, the government continued to set targets and use the data to report on health outcomes. Performance management of providers also remained part and parcel of the health framework.

Moreover, patient choice, professional power and localism, which imply moving responsibility down to the local tier of government, essentially aim at trying to make the public sector more efficient and are part of a rationing process. The reforms that took place in 2012 were made to cut costs since the PCTs were seen as more expensive to run than CCGs. Priority has thus been given to cutting costs and making efficiency gains, which are key aspects of NPM. For instance, a Quality, Innovation Productivity and Prevention (QIPP) programme was enacted in 2010 with a view to saving £20 billion by 2015 (Department of Health, 2010). The 2010-2015 government extended the use of PbR to promote quality and clinical effectiveness with the introduction of best-practice tariffs. Best-practice tariffs pay providers according to the actual cost of best clinical practice rather than the national average cost of care.

In addition, the contracting out of services to the private sector is still promoted via the CCGs. The latter are in fact actively encouraged to put services out to tender, in order to encourage non-NHS providers to bid in order to take over the running of services in a particular area. Indeed, seven out of ten NHS contracts have been taken on by private companies or institutions (NHS Support Federation, 2017). It would therefore seem that NPM techniques are still very much a feature of public healthcare provision in England.

In essence, despite some incremental changes in the post-NPM period, it is clear that there has been increased emphasis on market-based governance mechanisms, purchasing and providing, contracting out and on choice for patients. The essential problem of building on NPM reforms is that health is being led by political aspirations rather than public good principles. Moreover, performance indicators are ill-adapted to health. The diagnosis and treatment of health conditions and their outputs are complex and differ from one patient to the next, which makes measuring outputs and applying performance indicators tricky. Moreover, the continuation of NPM techniques which focus on private sector management practices has overturned the public service ethos. It has also weakened trade unions and collective bargaining because of contracting out, local employment contracts and individual performance-related pay.

In addition, it is not clear whether the quality of health services has actually gained from NPM and post-NPM governance. The OECD reported, after the series of reforms to the NHS, that the UK is very much middle-of-the-road for health outcomes. It may have an above average life expectancy rate, but primary prevention[5] is often seen to be neglected because of the overriding emphasis on targets and the reliance on new providers from the private sector (OECD, 2015). In addition, recent reports from the Care Quality Commission (CQC) and other sources (BBC, Patients' Association, etc.) have revealed problems in the care provided in hospital and long-stay hospital residence.

Additional cuts to local authority budgets mean that, although the government has given more power to local government to manage health, they have not given the authorities the means to ensure high standards in health and social care.

It is thus evident from our analysis of the reconfiguration and reform of health services that there has been a clear change in the role of the state and shifting forms of governance. Yet Ham underlines that the evolution of health policy under NPM shows how politicians were at the heart of the reforms of the NHS. The government was clearly at the centre of changes and reforms in health policy (Ham, 2009). Ham argues that throughout the reform process, health bodies and pressure groups within the sector were excluded from negotiations, which shows the force of the political executive to make radical changes to health policy. The State still plays a central role in ensuring that the NHS remains a public service free at the point of use. However, part of the internal management of public services has passed to external managers, private commissioners and arm's length bodies[6] with an increasing role for the market for service provision. Decision making has been devolved from central to local and regional bodies, but the state still remains the principal regulator of service providers and sets the ideological direction of the NHS. As Rothgang (2010) concludes, the role of the state has changed but is not necessarily less important in the governance of health services.

NPM BEYOND THE UK

Yet NPM reforms are not unique to the UK. From the 1980s onwards, a series of European directives encouraged the liberalisation of public sectors and notably the electricity sector, postal services, public transport, etc. The contracting out of services such as hospital catering, rubbish collection and highway maintenance has now become common in France, Germany and Spain. The European Union has sought to go further with market reforms of public services. For example, the European Union tried to implement the Bolkenstein Directive in order to create a single market for all services, including those provided by government. It failed to be implemented, but there is increasing pressure to assimilate public services in the private sector. In addition, the EU introduced new terminology 'services of general interest' rather than public services. The Commission explained that it was done to fulfil citizens' demands with an open and competitive market as the main instrument. Hence it is about 'serving the public'. This is clearly in line with

Figure 2. Changes to the structure of the NHS in England: On the creation of the NHS in 1948
Source: House of Commons, 2014

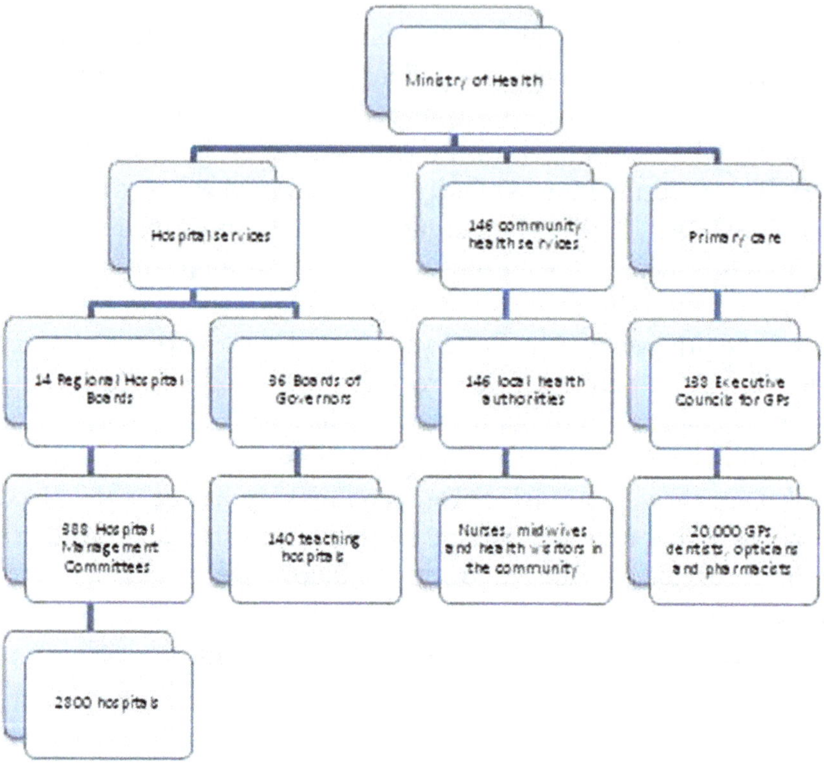

new public management which promotes consumer sovereignty and greater choice for public services. The WTO and the General Agreement on Trade in Services have also tried to open public services to trade, as have cross-regional agreements which will be covered in Chapter 8. What is remarkable, however, in the case of the UK, and more specifically England after devolution, is the extent to which the public sector has been transformed. As Pierson points out, very few cases in OECD countries show such radical changes as the UK (Pierson, 1996). In particular, two select countries, France and Norway introduced more moderate forms of NPM than Britain.

Figure 3. Changes to the structure of the NHS in England: Pre-April 2013 Structure
Source: House of Commons, 2014

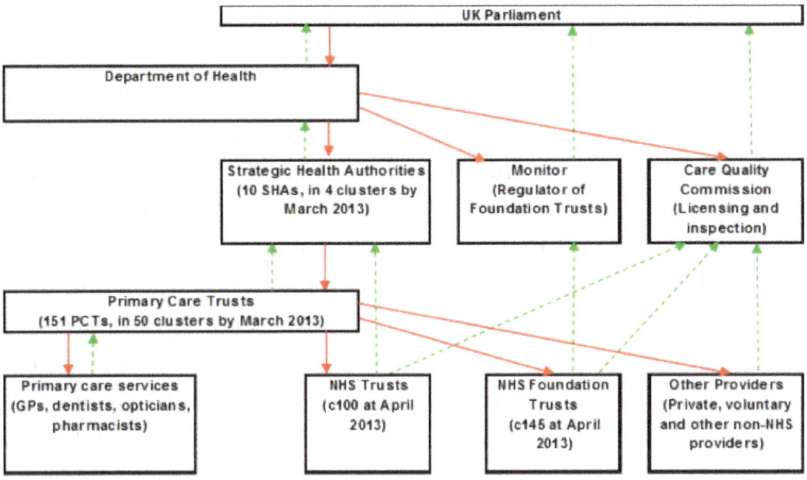

Figure 4. Changes to the structure of the NHS in England: Post April 13 structure
Source: House of Commons, 2014

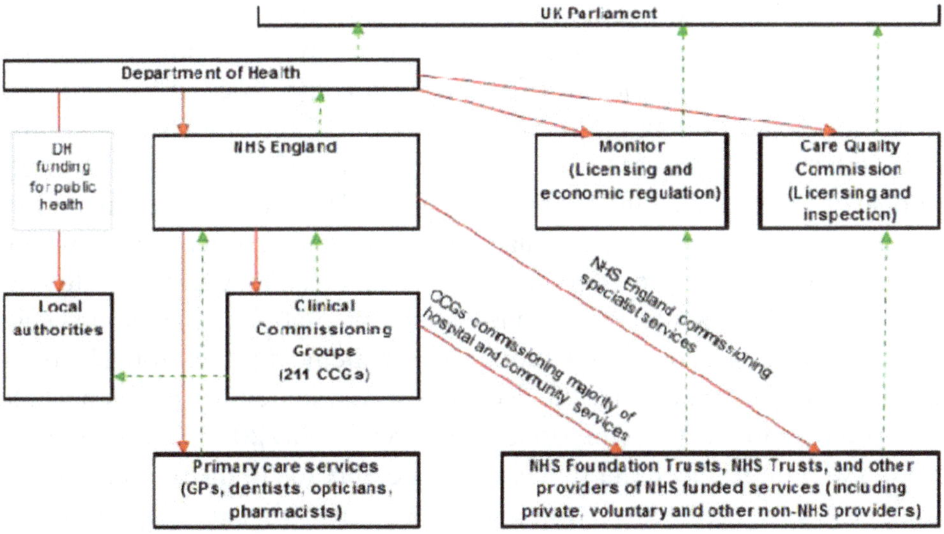

New Public Management in France

Market governance would appear to have been less significant in France than in the UK. Nevertheless, a wave of agentification took place in this country in the 1990s, especially following the Juppé reforms of 1996 and led to the creation of regional hospital agencies. These agencies thus took over some of the responsibilities from the Ministry of Health in determining health priorities at regional level. Such reforms were instrumental in introducing management practices within the French healthcare system, with for example multi-year performance contracts for care providers. A National Accreditation and Evaluation Agency and a High Authority on Health were also introduced to monitor performance in the same way as health authorities in England. The creation of Diagnostic Related Groups (DRGs) in 2004, has also been said to draw on two basic principles of NPM: firstly, it led to a split in funding from the government and care provision by hospitals and, secondly, it introduced a degree of incentivisation and competition for patients because care providers' income thus became related to patient volume. Previously, funding from central government had depended on patient length of stay, demographics and hospital bargaining power. Since the enactment of this law, poor performing units within hospitals with high costs or few patients have had to make changes to improve profitability or have been ordered to close. While hospitals were previously often run by municipalities and according to town or local priorities, targets are now centrally-led and often do not take into account the specificities of the region. Contract-based management between regional health agencies and hospitals is also said to have laid the foundations for quasi-markets which define financing grants and activity targets, patient volumes, etc. for care providers. However, France is not considered to have gone as far as the UK with quasi-market implementation in the public health service because of strong opposition from the medical profession. Hospitals do not just depend on DRGs, but also receive supplementary payments to be able to fund public services missions. Moreover, in May 2012, *Le Plan Hôpital* reforms were introduced in France, which notably led to the reintegration of physicians into hospital governance and a focus on quality and responsiveness to move away from the previous market-oriented reforms (Simonet, 2014).

Health Sector Reforms in Norway

Despite the tradition of a generous welfare state, Norway also brought in reforms in the 1990s in line with NPM. For example, unitary management systems, performance measurement models and a free patient choice model were introduced into the Norwegian public healthcare system. An activity-based funding system based on diagnosis and quality control was also part and parcel of the reforms. However, perhaps the most significant NPM reform in Norway was the transformation of hospitals into enterprises. Five regional health enterprises were created in 2002. They were independent entities with boards and managing directors and were encouraged to administer healthcare according to the market model. The discourse was very similar to that of the UK in that managerial processes were expected to enhance efficiency within hospitals. Yet the control still remained at the centre because it was the Ministry of Health who appointed the board members. What has emerged in practice, owing to the fairly generous social regime in Norway, is that many of these enterprises are actually controlled and directed by government and remain centred on the traditional public service model (Christensen & Laegreid, 2006).

The UK's national health system has thus been aligned far more to a market model than many European countries. However, this is perhaps not so evident for the service user who still receives universal health coverage.

ORGANISATION OF HEALTHCARE DELIVERY TODAY

Indeed, despite the move towards market governance, the NHS still provides care free at the point of use today. The NHS provides for preventive services such as screening, immunisation and vaccination, inpatient and outpatient hospital care and drugs, physician services, inpatient and outpatient drugs, dental care which is deemed clinically necessary, mental healthcare, palliative care, some long-term care, rehabilitation, physiotherapy and home visits. However, the volume and scope depends on local decision making bodies which are nevertheless supposed to follow the recommendations of NICE (in England, Wales and Northern Ireland) or Health Improvement in Scotland. There are some charges for prescription drugs in England, although NHS hospital drugs are free. Scotland, Wales and Northern Ireland abolished prescription charges altogether after devolution in all public healthcare settings. NHS dentistry, besides essential care, is subject to co-payments. However, children under 18 and in full-time education, people aged 60 or over, low income and pregnant women are exempted from prescription drug and dental co-payments. Vision tests are also free for the aforementioned groups (Thorlby & Arora, 2015).

GP Practices

Primary care can be defined as healthcare provided in the community for people making an initial approach to a medical practitioner or clinic for advice or treatment. This care is provided through general practitioners (GPs) across the UK. Secondary care can be defined as medical care provided by a specialist or facility upon referral by a primary care physician. In order to receive this care, patients must consult their GP first. In 2018, there were 150,000 doctors across the four nations of the UK (Rolewicz & Palmer, 2019). Patients must register with a local practice of their choice, but this may be difficult if the practice is already full and this will thus limit their choice. There are also a number of walk-in centres in some localities whereby patients do not have to register to receive primary care services. Part of the work, which is often the remit of GPs in other countries, is carried out by nurses employed in most GP practices. They monitor patients for blood pressure and/or provide minor treatments. In total 320,000 nurses and midwives work across hospital, community and primary healthcare settings (Rolewicz & Palmer, 2019).

Outpatient Specialist Care

Specialist care is highly regulated and monitored in the UK. The vast majority of specialists are salaried employees in NHS hospitals. The CCGs pay hospitals to cover these outpatient consultations but at structured and nationally determined rates. Specialists can charge more however if they set up private practitioners within designated NHS hospital wards or in private hospitals. Patients may choose the hospital unit and specialist team depending on availability (Thorlby & Arora, 2015).

Hospitals

Hospitals in England are run by trusts or foundation trusts and regulated by NHS Improvement. Hospital trusts are often encouraged to apply for foundation status because it effectively gives them more autonomy to provide services in the local community. Although they remain public institutions free at the point of use, they have more freedom to manage their budget independently than regular trusts but they still remain accountable to Parliament. Both types of trusts must contract with the local CCG in order to provide services. Services are reimbursed following a nationally determined diagnosis-related group (DRG) rate, taking into account the majority of the costs. Some rates are made by services (emergency care, elective surgery, etc.) or according to long-term hospital care services, such as diabetes units. Both NHS public and private hospital services in England are monitored by NHS Improvement and the Care Quality Commission (CQC), but private providers are free to charge the rates they choose. NHS Improvement and the CQC are also responsible for monitoring and regulating NHS services. NHS Improvement also sets prices for NHS-funded services, it helps mitigate against the disruption of local services if commissioners meet financial difficulties. The CQC is responsible for monitoring, inspecting and regulating the safety and security of services provided by both health and social care actors in hospitals, dentist surgeries, ambulances, care homes, and within the provision of domiciliary care. As for the surveillance of public health, the department of Health sets the policies and Public Health England leads and advises local authorities on how to implement public health policies (National Assembly for Wales, 2015). It is difficult to calculate accurately the number of hospitals in England, but all acute, mental, specialist and community hospitals are governed by trusts. There are currently 223 trusts in England, many of which are in charge of running more than just one hospital. In Wales, seven local health boards and four NHS trusts run hospitals. In Northern Ireland, there are six hospital trusts. In Scotland, 14 territorial boards run the hospitals.

Long-term Care and Social Support

The majority of long-term care is provided by local authorities in England and the private sector, even for patients with underlying healthcare needs. Only people with very specific medical needs which require skilled nursing will be eligible for full NHS coverage. There are approximately 5,500 providers and 11,300 care homes for the elderly and physically disabled across the UK. Approximately 95% of beds are provided by the independent sector, both for profit and charitable providers. Assets need to be very low in order to benefit from full social care. The threshold is £23,250 in England and

Northern Ireland, £26,500 in Scotland, and £30,000 in Wales to receive free care in care homes, domiciliary care, or other types of care. In the UK, 41% of residents in care homes fund themselves (self-funders) and 49% receive Local Authority (LA) funding (around a quarter of these pay top-ups). The NHS in the four legislatures covers end-of-life palliative care at patients' homes, in hospices (usually run by charitable organisations), in care homes, or in hospitals (Competition and Markets Authority (CMA), 2017).

CONCLUSION

Since the NPM reforms, ushered in by the New Right government in 1979 onwards, it is clear that market governance has been central in the delivery of health services in the UK, especially in England, for the latter period of reforms. The move towards using private sector techniques to run public health services has been reinforced and been taken much further than in many other European countries. Yet the NHS still provides a healthcare system free at the point of use which covers approximately 80% of all healthcare costs for individuals residing in the UK. However, the cost of maintaining such a system has led to a number of initiatives, including greater involvement of the private sector in the running of the NHS, as will be described in the next chapter.

REFERENCES

Aaron, H. J., Schwartz, W. B., & Cox, C. (2005). *Can we say no? The challenge of rationing healthcare*. Brookings Institution Press.

Abel-Smith, B. (1978). *National health service: The first thirty years*. HMSO.

Bacon, R., & Eltis, W. (1976). *Britain's economic problem: Too few producers*. Macmillan.

BBC News. (2002, July 11). *NHS history: the 70s*. Retrieved September 8, 2018, from http://news.bbc.co.uk/2/hi/programmes/the_service/2120283.stm

Bevir, M., & Rhodes, R. A. W. (2003). *Interpreting British governance*. Routledge.

Buchanan, J. M., & Tullock, G. (1962). *The calculus of consent*. Liberty Fund.

Christensen, T., & Laegreid, P. (2006). *Autonomy and regulation: Coping with agencies in the modern state.* Edward Elgar.

Clark, D. (1996). Open government in Britain: Discourse and practice. *Public Money & Management, 16*(1), 23–30. doi:10.1080/09540969609387905

Clarke, E., Leaver, L., & Gilbert, B. J. (2015, June). Morality not markets: A manifesto for the NHS; Response to Pollock, Frith, and Cox. *International Journal of Health Policy and Management, 4*(6), 409–410. doi:10.15171/ijhpm.2015.78 PMID:26029904

Clarke, J. (2007). It's not like shopping: Citizens, consumers, and the reform of public services. In M. Bevir & F. Trentmann (Eds.), *Governance, consumers and citizens: Agency and resistance in contemporary politics* (pp. 97–118). Palgrave MacMillan. doi:10.1057/9780230591363_5

Competition and Market's Authority (CMA). (2017, November 30). *Care home's market study.* London: Crown. Retrieved April 5, 2020, from https://assets.publishing.service.gov.uk/media/5a1fdf30e5274a750b82533a/care-homes-market-study-final-report.pdf

Cutler, T. (2003). Dangerous yardstick? Early cost estimates and the politics of financial management in the first decade of the National Health Service. *Medical History, 47*(2), 217–238. doi:10.1017/S0025727300056726 PMID:12754765

Department of Health. (1992). *The health of the nation – a strategy for health in England.* HMSO.

Department of Health. (1997). The new NHS: Modern, dependable. CM 3807. HMSO.

Department of Health. (1998, July 1). *A first class service: Quality in the new NHS.* HSC 1998/113. Crown.

Department of Health. (2010). *Equity and excellence: Liberating the NHS.* HMSO.

Department of Health and Social Security. (1989). *Working for patients.* HMSO.

Dillow, C. (2007). *The end of politics: New Labour and the folly of managerialism.* Harriman House.

Dorey, P. (2015). The legacy of thatcherism – Public sector reform. L'héritage du thatchérisme, Observatoire de la Société Britannique, 17, 33-60.

Dorling, D. (2013). *Unequal health: The scandal of our times*. The Policy Press. doi:10.2307/j.ctt1t891pj

Enroth, H. (2014). Governance: The art of governing after governmentality. *European Journal of Social Theory*, *17*(1), 60–76. doi:10.1177/1368431013491818

Executive, N. H. S. (1999). *The NHS performance assessment framework*. NHS.

Gorsky, M. (2008). The British National Health Service 1948–2008: A review of the historiography. *Social History of Medicine*, *21*(3), 437–460. doi:10.1093hm/hkn064

Gregory, S., Dixon, A., & Ham, C. (2012). *Health policy under the Coalition government: A mid-term assessment*. The King's Fund.

Griffiths, R. (1983). *NHS management inquiry*. Department of Health and Social Security.

Grimmeisen, S., & Frisina, L. (2010). The role of the state in the British healthcare system – between marketization and statism. In H. Rothgang, M. Cacace, L. Frisina, S. Grimmeisen, A. Schmid, & C. Wendt (Eds.), *The state and healthcare: Comparing OECD countries* (pp. 75–118). Palgrave Macmillan. doi:10.1057/9780230292345_5

Ham, C. (2009). *Health policy in Britain* (6th ed.). Palgrave Macmillan. doi:10.1007/978-1-137-01397-2

Hayek, F. (1944). *The road to serfdom*. Routledge Press.

Healthcare Commission. (2008). *Annual Report 2007/8*. Commission for Health, Audit and Inspection.

Hewitt, J. (2007). The impact of clinical governance on the professional autonomy and self-regulation of General Practitioners: Colonization or appropriation? In *Proceedings of new perspectives in the study of professionalism: Reconnecting professional organizations with professional organizations*. University of Waikoto.

Hodges, R., Wright, M., & Keasey, K. (1996). Corporate governance in the public services: Concepts and issues. *Public Money & Management*, *16*(2), 7–13. doi:10.1080/09540969609387915

Hood, C. (1991). A Public Management for all Seasons. *Public Administration*, *69*(2), 3–19. doi:10.1111/j.1467-9299.1991.tb00779.x

House of Commons. (2015). *Health Committee. NHS continuing care. Sixth report of session 2014–2015*. The Stationery Office.

Katsamunska, P. (2016). The concept of governance and public governance theories. *Economic Alternatives*, *2*, 133–141.

Klein, R. (2006). *The new politics of the NHS: From creation to reinvention*. Radcliffe Publishing.

Kouzmin, A., Loffler, E., Klages, H., & Korac-Kakabadse, N. (1999). Benchmarking and performance measurement in public sectors: Towards learning for agency effectiveness. *International Journal of Public Sector Management*, *12*(2), 121–129. doi:10.1108/09513559910263462

Lapsley, I. (1994). Market mechanisms and the management of healthcare. The UK model and experience. *International Journal of Public Sector Management*, *7*(6), 15–25. doi:10.1108/09513559410070551

Le Grand, J. (2003). *Motivation, agency and public policy: Of knights and knaves, pawns and queens*. Oxford University Press. doi:10.1093/0199266999.001.0001

Marin, B., & Mayntz, R. (1991). Introduction: Studying Policy Networks. In B. Marin & R. Mayntz (Eds.), Empirical evidence and theoretical considerations (pp. 11-23). Campus.

Marsh, D., & Rhodes, R. A. W. (1992). Policy communities and issue networks. Beyond typology. In D. Marsh & R. A. W. Rhodes (Eds.), *Policy networks in British government* (pp. 249–268). Clarendon Press. doi:10.1093/acprof:oso/9780198278528.003.0011

National Audit Office. (2017). *A short guide to selected health arm's length bodies*. NAO.

Nelson, E., & Nikolov, K. (2001). *UK inflation in the 1970s and 1980s: The role of output gap mismeasurement*. Bank of England. Retrieved September 10, 2018, from file:///D:/V10866/Documents/recentchanges/healthpublication/2020versionNHS/uk-inflation-in-the-1970s-and-1980s-the-role-of-output-gap-mismeasurement.pdf

OECD. (2013). *Health at a glance*. OECD.

OECD. (2015). *Health at a glance*. OECD.

Offe, C. (2009). Governance: An "Empty Signifier". *Constellations (Oxford, England), 16*(4), 550–562. doi:10.1111/j.1467-8675.2009.00570.x

Pierson, P. (1996, January). The new politics of the welfare state. *World Politics, 48*(2), 143–179. doi:10.1353/wp.1996.0004

Pollock, A. M. (2004). *NHS plc: The privatisation of our healthcare*. Verso.

Rhodes, R. A. W. (1997). *Understanding governance*. Open University Press.

Roberts, R. (2016). *When Britain went bust: The 1976 IMF crisis*. OMFIF Press.

Rolewicz, L., & Palmer, B. (2019). *The NHS workforce in numbers*. Nuffield Trust. Retrieved June 20, 2019, from https://www.nuffieldtrust.org.uk/resource/the-nhs-workforce-in-numbers

Rothgang, H. (2010). The converging role of the state in OECD healthcare systems. In H. Rothgang, M. Cacace, L. Frisina, S. Grimmeisen, A. Schmid, & C. Wendt (Eds.), *The state and healthcare: Comparing OECD countries* (pp. 237–247). Palgrave Macmillan. doi:10.1057/9780230292345_8

Scally, G., & Donaldson, L. (1998, July 4). The NHS's 50 anniversary. Clinical governance and the drive for quality improvement in the new NHS in England. *British Medical Journal, 317*(7150), 61–65. doi:10.1136/bmj.317.7150.61 PMID:9651278

Simonet, D. (2014). Assessment of new public management in healthcare: The French case. *Health Research Policy and Systems, 12*(1), 57. doi:10.1186/1478-4505-12-57 PMID:25283813

Smith, P. (Ed.). (2002). *Measuring up: Improving health system performance in OECD countries*. OECD.

Social Market Foundation. (2005). *To the point: A blueprint for good targets*. SMF.

Thorlby, R., & Arora, S. (2015). *The English healthcare system*. Nuffield Trust. Retrieved July 6, 2018, from https://international.commonwealthfund.org/countries/england/

Wanless, D. (2002). *Securing our future health: Taking a long-term view*. HMSO.

Wanless, D. (2004). *Securing good health for the whole population*. HMSO.

Webster, C. (2002). *The National Health Service – A political history*. Oxford University Press.

Whitaker, P. (2015, March 5). How Labour broke the NHS – and why Labour must fix it. *New Statesman*. Retrieved July 7, 2018, from https://www.newstatesman.com/politics/2015/03/how-labour-broke-nhs-and-why-labour-must-fix-it

ENDNOTES

1 Public choice theory is an economic theory developed from the study of taxation and public spending. It implies using economic tools and applying them to problems of political science.

2 The tenets were also visible elsewhere: in the education sector, for example.

3 For a more detailed discussion of localism, see Chapter 5.

4 The NHS Constitution, first published in 2009, sets out rights for patients, the general public and staff. It also underlines the responsibilities of the latter to ensure a fair and effective provision of NHS health services.

5 Primary Prevention relates to measures taken to prevent a disease or injury before it occurs.

6 The National Audit Office (2017) underlines that health arm's length bodies fall into five categories: executive agencies (part of the Department of Health), special health authorities (subject to the direction of the Secretary of State, for example the NHS Counter Fraud Authority created in 2017-18), executive non-departmental public bodies, advisory non-departmental public bodies and expert committees.

Chapter 2
Financial Governance and the NHS

ABSTRACT

Faced with significant difficulties to meet financial costs owing to increased demand for healthcare, National Health Service (NHS) organisations are looking to maintain tight financial control and reduce expenditure where possible. Significant price hikes in essential medicines can also raise challenges to the supply of necessary drugs for the population. The NHS continues to supply healthcare free at the point of use and any attempts to introduce charges remain unpopular. There have been a number of ways in which providers endeavour to reduce costs: rationalisation (reduction of services or certain costly drugs) or through increasing the role of private providers in healthcare provision. This chapter thus reviews the funding challenges the NHS is currently facing and how financial governance is evolving to meet those challenges.

INTRODUCTION

The previous chapter described the move since the 1980s towards a market-oriented approach in the NHS. The major driving force behind such fundamental changes was the need to make savings, faced with ever-increasing health demands. Indeed, health services in the UK have been under significant pressure to keep costs down. Longevity, the retirement of the baby generations of the 1940s and the expected impact of the retirement of the 1960s baby boomers

DOI: 10.4018/978-1-7998-3928-6.ch002

has meant that there are greater health demands. In addition, medical and technological progress has resulted in rising drug and medical device costs. The financial crisis of 2008, the ensuing recession and low growth have also put extra pressure on government budgets. The Covid-19 pandemic, which has put significant pressure on health systems around the world in 2020, will most probably result in further financial difficulties for healthcare providers despite support from the British government. This chapter will thus describe those financial pressures in detail. It will then look at a number of solutions which have been envisaged to sustain healthcare provision, including the privatisation of some areas of healthcare provision.

FINANCIAL PRESSURES IN THE NHS

Financial pressures on the health service have continued to rise in recent years and are expected to continue in the future. In 50 years, the Organisation for National Statistics (ONS) projects that there will be an additional 8.6 million people over the age of 65 and by 2030 one in five people will be 65 or over (ONS, 2018). The average cost of health and social care for the elderly is six times that for 16-44 year olds, which obviously puts significant pressure on national healthcare systems (Barker, 2014). The same applies to the cost of surgery and technological progress which will cause costs to rise. However, more efficient use of technology and the development of drugs such as statins to control cholesterol should lower the need for heart surgery. Better chronic disease management should also reduce the cost of emergency hospital admissions. But overall costs have risen substantially and will continue to increase because of rising health demands. Staff costs also continue to rise and more specialised skills are needed and technology cannot replace the need for qualified clinicians.

Public healthcare in the UK is financed by taxation. The total amount of taxation allocated to the NHS is voted annually according to clearly defined government priorities, projections and economic growth and the government's revenue position. Healthcare takes up a sizeable portion of the UK's public expenditure which has risen rapidly since the creation of the NHS in 1948 from 11.4 billion in the first year of its operation to 152.9 billion in 2018/9 (Harker, 2019). Growth in health expenditure has thus outpaced GDP growth over the last few decades. Funding is allocated across the four nations of the

UK. In 2018/9, expenditure per head on health services was the highest in Northern Ireland (£2,436 per head) and the lowest in England (£2,269 per head) (Harker, 2019). In 2019/20, planned spending just for England was £139.3 billion with the majority of this budget covering day-to-day costs such as salaries and medicines. The remainder was devoted to capital spending on buildings and equipment (£7 billion) (Harker, 2019).

Given the funding crisis, a number of measures have been taken in an attempt to increase efficiency. In England the Quality, Innovation, Productivity and Prevention initiative was introduced in 2011 aiming for £20 billion of savings over the period to 2015 in order to maintain the delivery of high quality services (The Health Foundation, 2015). This amounted to a target of 4% efficiency gains a year. Given that NHS productivity growth averaged 0.5% per year until 2010, this target seems rather ambitious. Between 2010 and 2012, public sector pay was frozen to help keep NHS cost pressures down. Tightening of contract negotiations and tariffs by hospitals negotiated by Primary Care Trusts (PCTs) and then Clinical Commissioning Groups (CCGs) was expected to make an extra 40% in savings. However, since these efficiency gains were aiming at constraining inputs rather than increasing outputs, efficiency gains could only be seen to be temporary and have limited effects. It has been reported that NHS productivity even fell by about 1% between 2012-13 and 2013-14 after the introduction of this initiative (The Health Foundation, 2015). Despite the introduction of methods to keep costs down and to evaluate cost effectiveness with the introduction of performance indicators, costs have continued to rise.

According to the Institute of Fiscal Studies, the NHS suffered its worst financial crisis ever in 2015/6. At the end of the 2015/16 fiscal year, NHS providers and commissioners reported a deficit of £1.85 billion (unaudited) (NHS England, 2016), which represents three times that recorded in the previous year and the largest deficit in the history of the NHS. While health expenditure was ring-fenced, despite the introduction of austerity measures in England in 2010, the budget for the NHS was originally set relatively low and predicted to increase by £8.4 billion in real terms by 2020-21. This is comparatively low from an international perspective and insufficient to make up for the shortfall in funding. In a letter to *The Guardian*, former chief executive of NHS England, Sir David Nicholson, and a number of high ranking General Practitioners (GPs) and academics, deplored the fact that "Our health service is now exhibiting the symptoms of a very ill patient, and it is our firmly held belief that a different course of treatment is needed if we are to reverse early-stage terminal decline" (Campbell, 2015, para. 4). They continued: "The NHS is in dire financial straits and this is beginning to undermine the health of our nation" (Campbell, 2015, para. 6). Dr Mark Porter, chairman of the British Medical Association (BMA), did not diagnose the worst outcome for the NHS, but he argued that the NHS was facing "unprecedented" challenges and "without the investment needed to secure the future of services, the quality of patient care would be at risk, and an NHS true to its founding principles" would be very much under threat (Campbell, 2015, para. 12).

Ahead of the 2017 Autumn statement, researchers at three health think tanks: The King's Fund, Nuffield Trust and the Health Foundation, reported that the estimated rise in total health spending in England (from £123.8 billion in 2017/18 to £128.4 billion by the end of the parliament in 2022/23) was much less than the amount necessary to maintain current standards of care and meet rising demand (The King's Fund, 2017). In July 2018, the government pledged a new five-year funding deal for England increasing health spending by 3.4% on average for the period 2019/20 to 2023/24. However, the funding increase only applied to NHS England services and not the overall Department of Health and Social Care budget. Thus it excluded important areas in need of extra financing so, in September 2019, the government announced further increases to cover capital investment, education and training of the NHS workforce. Nevertheless, the overall average increase of the Department of Health and Social Care budget (2.9% between 2019/20 and 2020/21) is lower than the long run average trend. According to the King's Fund, the funding increases will only ease current pressures and not lead to the transformation of services or better healthcare delivery (The King's Fund, 2020).

There is also significant pressure on health budgets in the localities because of changing governance patterns. Since 2013, pursuant to the Health and Social Care Act of 2012, public health responsibilities (and notably ill health prevention), which had been part of the NHS, have been transferred to local government in England. Local government services, including those relating to health, have not been ring-fenced from the cuts. Local authority health budgets were cut further, by 3.9% a year, in addition to the £200 million that was already taken from the 2015/16 budget (HM Treasury, 2015).

While UK health expenditure remains above the OECD average, it is still lower than many of its EU counterparts. According to the OECD, total spending on health, including private spending, amounted to 9.8% of the UK's share of GDP in 2018 compared to 11.2% in both France and Germany (OECD, 2019). Government funding on health spending is also lower in the UK compared with many of its European competitors. In 2018, government

Figure 1. Health expenditure as a share of GDP, 2018 (or nearest year) in OECD countries
Source: OECD Health Statistics (2019), WHO Global Health Expenditure Database

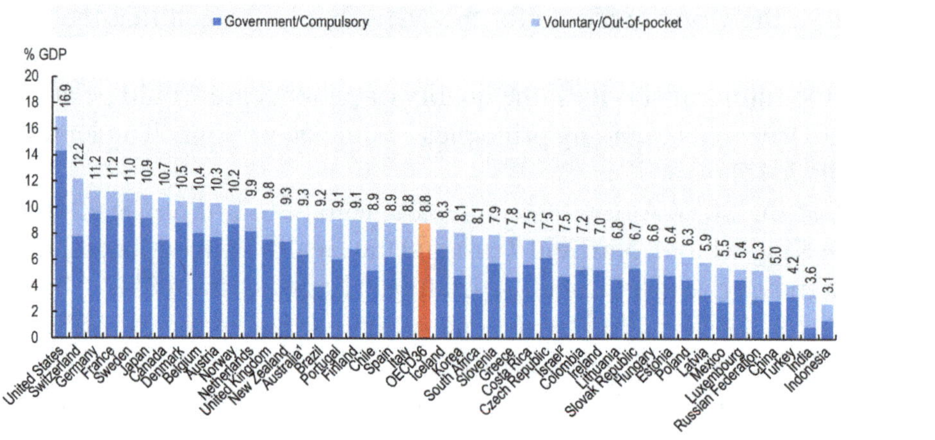

Note: Expenditure excludes investments, unless otherwise stated.
1. Australian expenditure estimates exclude all expenditure for residential aged care facilities in welfare (social) services.
2. Includes investments

spending on health amounted to approximately 8% of GDP, compared to 9% of GDP in France and 10% of GDP in Germany (OECD, 2019).

However, the situation in Scotland is somewhat different, with per capita expenditure almost 10% higher than in England (Camp-Pietrain, 2019). Indeed, 43% of the Scottish budget is spent on the NHS. While social deprivation and geographical disperson may explain the need to have greater expenditure, in Scotland it is also political will. In the seventies, faced with separatist tensions, the British government devised a formula (the Barnett Formula) guaranteeing the increase of the Scottish budget, indexed on the public expenditure for England. The sum obtained was managed in Scotland, first by the Secretary of State for Scotland and then after 1999 by the Scottish government, which, free to arbitrate between their areas of competence, have given priority to health (Camp-Pietrain, 2019). Yet despite a greater outlay, Scotland is also suffering from significant pressures on funding similar to other administrations. For all the four nations of the UK, some of the significant pressure on the budget comes from the cost of providing drugs.

Price Escalation in the Pharmaceutical Sector

The rising cost of medicines to the NHS is cause for concern. A study by the King's Fund reported that the total estimated cost of NHS spending on medicines in England had increased from £13 billion in 2010/11 to £17.4 billion in 2016/7, which represents an average growth of 5% a year (NHS Digital, 2017; Ewbank, Omojomolo, Sullivan, & McKenna, 2018). This is a faster rate of growth than the growth of the total NHS budget over the same period and is mainly due to spending in the hospital sector. The dramatic increase in prices described can be explained by the increase in the average cost per prescription item from £8.26 in 1996 to £10.96 in 2006 for hospital prescriptions (NHS information Centre, 2007; Ewbank et al., 2018). Nevertheless, these figures overstate the real price of medicines because they are the official ex-factory prices. In practice, confidential discounts are accorded to the NHS. Moreover, the NHS actually receives a rebate from the pharmaceutical industry as part of the Pharmaceutical Price Regulation Scheme (PPRS) and this is not included in the price.

The NHS has developed a tight framework to control escalation of prices. The policy on medicines aims to balance the competing goals of giving patients prompt access to effective treatments, to incentivise the pharmaceutical sector to develop new products and ensure affordability of medicines for the NHS. Before they can be administered to patients, pharmaceutical products must undergo regulatory approval either by the European Medicines Agency or by the UK medicines regulator (Medicines and Healthcare Products Regulatory Agency) to monitor their safety and effectiveness. After regulatory approval, the National Institute for Health and Care (NICE), in consultation with the Department of Health and Social Care, then determine whether they can be provided by the NHS in terms of their clinical and cost effectiveness. In particular, NICE uses Quality-Adjusted Life Years (QALYs) to measure the health gain that a product offers, and thus a calculation of the product's Incremental Cost-Effectiveness Ratio (ICER) is calculated to see how much the treatment costs (Poole, 2008). The Competition and Market Authority (CMA) will intervene if anti-competition policies are practiced, such as for example the fine imposed on Pfizer and Flynne Pharma in 2016 for hiking the price of an anti-epilepsy product, phenytoin.

The pricing system in England is complex and quite exceptional in advanced health systems because it uses a number of different instruments to influence prices of different categories of medicine. The Pharmaceutical

Price Regulations Scheme is a voluntary agreement between the Department of Health and Social Care and the Association of the British Pharmaceutical Industry (ABPI) (of which 94% of British pharmaceutical companies are a member), which aims to control expenditure on branded medication. Companies must provide cost-neutral access to drugs which means that any product introduced must be offset by another process to reduce costs (Department of Health and Association of the British Pharmaceutical Industry, 2013). If sales exceed the agreed level of growth, the industry has to make payments to the Department of Health and Social Care. Constraints on medicines and these pricing mechanisms means that UK spending on medicines was in the lower half of 15 EU countries in 2015 (OECD, 2017).

The NHS has a number of other policies to reduce the cost of medicine, namely the widespread use of cheaper generic versions of drugs and biosimilars (generics for biological products), etc. A budget impact test for new products has also been introduced whereby any new products that cost more than £20 million a year are subject to commercial negotiation with a delay clause if a negotiation cannot be reached (Timmins, 2017). However, the problematic issue is for new medicines, since it has been estimated that 20% of new medicines cost more than £20 million (Timmins, 2017). Access to new high-profile treatments such as hepatitis C have been delayed as a result (Boseley, 2015).

In addition, the agreement that the NHS has with pharmaceutical companies has come under scrutiny because it is argued that it enables the pharmaceutical industry to make profits at the expense of ensuring value for money in the delivery of NHS services (Claxton, 2007). While there do seem to be restrictions on the amount pharmaceutical companies can charge the NHS, it would seem the close relationship between pharmaceutical companies and NHS hospitals and CCGs might sometimes also represent a conflict of interest. For example, a Freedom of Information request (FOI) identified that at least 36 CCGs had been involved in medicines management programmes financed directly or indirectly by the drug industry. More than 1,000 GP practices had accepted funding from the drugs company Bayer to finance 'medicines optimisation work' for new anticoagulant drugs for patients with atrial fibrillation (McCarthney, 2015). In essence, such partnerships should help to provide safe administration of drugs. The argument is that although drug companies make a profit, they also ensure safe use because the professionals are paid to educate NHS staff and patients on how to use the drugs. However, a parliamentary inquiry found that oversight of the pharmaceutical industry had been lax and that a profit relationship had developed between health administrators and pharmaceutical companies, which was against the public interest. The inquiry showed how drug promotion to professionals and patients groups was given priority by the pharmaceutical companies, the trial designs were inadequate and unsatisfactory trial results had been suppressed (McCarthney, 2015). Indeed, there is a suggestion that if the staff making the recommendations to take the drugs are actually being paid by the pharmaceutical company, this would seem to suggest a conflict of interest. David Watson from the Association of the British Pharmaceutical Industry (ABPI) argues that this is not necessarily the case and that the relationship needs to be well managed to avoid conflicts of interest: "We think it is a good thing all round, but there must always be clear governance and the nature of the agreement should also be transparent with the patient's best interest in mind" (McCarthney, 2015, p. 15). NHS bodies also encourage joint relationships. In a Memorandum of Understanding between NHS England, the Association of the British Pharmaceutical Industry (ABPI) and the British Generic Manufacturers Association (BGMA), it states:

NHS England and the pharmaceutical industry share mutual ambitions in improving health outcomes and quality of care. The transformational change needed across the health system will be delivered more effectively through effective co-operation and collaboration where we all stand to gain (NHS England, 2014, para. 6).

However, Dean Marshall from the BMA's General Practitioner's Committee argues that pharmaceutical companies should not have a close relationship with those making the clinical decisions to avoid clinicians being coerced into making decisions that are not in the best interest of the patient (McCartney, 2015).

Moreover, price hikes are still a sensitive issue in the NHS. The government had to ask the CMA to intervene and investigate allegations that Boots, a high street pharmacy chain, was overcharging the NHS for pain relieving mouthwash because it was taking advantage of a loophole which allows suppliers to set their own price for specials, which are unlicensed medicines (Morgan-Bentley, 2018). Overpricing has also been an issue with overseas suppliers. Indeed, the CMA accused Canadian firm Concordia of overcharging by £100m on a thyroid drug with the price per pack rising from £4.46 to £258 over 10 years. An investigation into drug price rises in the NHS showed that drug companies exploited loopholes to charge up to 2,358% more for medicines through 'debranding'. It means that while the rules governing branded drugs are strictly under control, Pharma companies re-categorise drugs. For example, phenytoin sodium capsules, used to treat epilepsy, increased from £2.3m to just over £50m in 2013 when it was debranded (Kollewe, 2017). The relationship between the pharmaceutical industry and NHS practitioners thus remains a complex one and requires careful governance in order for costs to be maintained.

FINANCIAL GOVERNANCE TO LIMIT COSTS

As providers and commissioners face deteriorating financial conditions because of rising costs, there has been an ever-increasing focus on financial governance, and how expenditure should be limited or alternative arrangements should be made to meet rising healthcare costs. This section will thus look at some suggested solutions and actual methods employed to drive down costs besides those which have already been outlined.

Introducing Fees or Taxes

The future funding of the NHS is a main concern because it is necessary to maintain a high level of care and meet the demands of an ageing population. Any discussion to introduce fees or privatise healthcare tends to meet with opposition. In general, the British population seems to be against privatisation. Indeed 84% of British people reported that they believed that the NHS should be run on a public basis (see figure 2). Even proposals to charge for GP visits, as in other European countries, do not seem to be popular.

Suggesting introducing charges within the public sector is thus controversial and problematic. Moreover, charges would also have to be applied to Accident and Emergency (A&E) services to avoid diversion problems and this could cause a lot of administrative pressure and extra costs. Therefore, it does not appear to be feasible to introduce charges in the NHS, except where units or clinics are completely privatised.

Another solution which has been put forward in an attempt to raise extra funds is hypothecation. This implies creating a specific tax which would go towards NHS funding. But earmarking taxes means that tax income can rise and fall and is therefore dependent on the economic cycle. Both Conservative and Labour chancellors have used tobacco tax to pay for part of NHS spending in the past. In 2002, Gordon Brown decided to add an

Figure 2. Public Opinion on Privatisation of the NHS

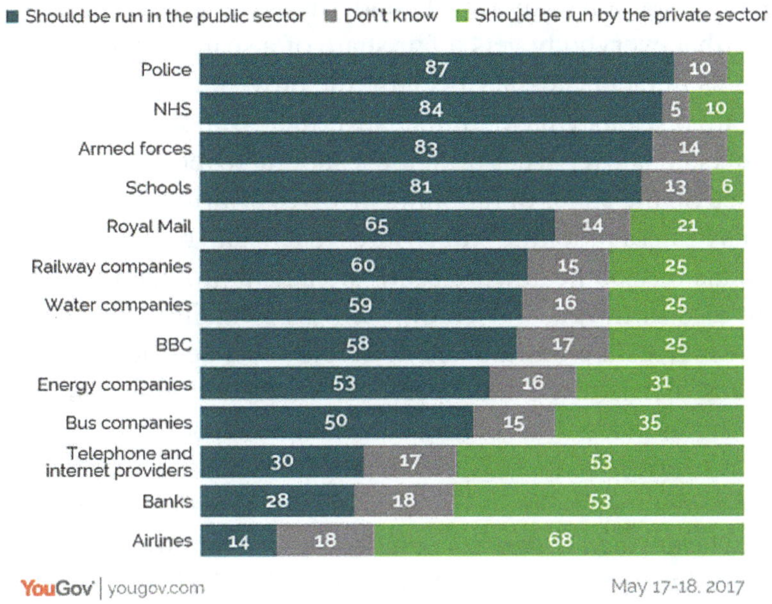

additional one percentage point on National Insurance to pay for a large increase in NHS funding. However, there was no subsequent information on how it contributed to the financing of the NHS. The King's Fund recommends the creation of a single, ring-fenced budget for health and social care and a unique commissioner, although certain observers contend that it could lead to greater privatisation of the health system. King's Fund researchers also suggest revisions to wealth taxation and reforms to inheritance tax to free up funds for the NHS (The King's Fund, 2015). In practice, since these solutions have not been implemented and finances are limited, a degree of rationing has taken place in the NHS.

Rationing Healthcare

Indeed, budgetary restraints have led to rationing of health services, which can have a significant impact on their delivery. A number of different but closely connected terms are used to define the attribution or restriction of resources: rationing, priority setting and resource allocation are often used interchangeably but with slightly different meanings (New, 1997). Rationing refers to the exclusion or denial of a service and withholding of resources. Priority setting relates to services or client groups and involves value judgments, whereas rationing is more technical and based on effectiveness (New, 1997). As Komaromy (2001) underlines, rationing is actually a way of ensuring that everybody gets a fair share of a scarce good. Some amount of rationing is in fact necessary because the provision and the ability to pay for healthcare obviously have limits. Nevertheless, policymakers do have a choice in decisions over what principles should govern and what priorities should be set. So the ethics of rationing involves priority setting and deciding whether this form of rationing still ensures that health remains a public good.

Individuals rely on healthcare professionals to provide them with better health, but also in the case of chronic illness to maintain levels of health. However, resources are limited and therefore must be prioritised according to need. This means using inter-personal subjective judgment as to what is best for the individual according to available resources. It also involves notions of cost-effectiveness. Clinicians will thus make a decision according to whether a treatment should be withheld because they need to save the resources to be devoted to another health case (Komaromy, 2001). Although rationing has always existed since the creation of the NHS, certain differences can be discerned between the rationing that has existed since the 1990s and rationing which predates this period. For example, Dr John Wilkinson, Consultant Dermatologist and Medical Director at South Bucks NHS Trust, contends that whereas prior to the 1990s reforms, rationing involved mainly medical decisions made on the basis of clinical assessment, today clinicians are rationing on a budgetary basis (Lenaghan, 1997). Ross Tristem, Director of the NHS Trust Federation, suggests that rationing became an issue in the 1990s because of targets and the Patients' Charter which means that there is more pressure to deliver and patients' expectations have thus become higher (Lenaghan, 1997). Indeed, needs have increased because of the huge progress in treatments and techniques available. Such progress has led to higher expectations on the part of patients.

According to Heginbotham (1997), rationing occurs either in a situation where there has been an under-provision of care or where demand is likely to continue to grow. It is thus considered to be necessary to restrict this growth. Rationing may also occur as a result of an innovation, for example if new equipment enables new service provision. Finally, limits to supply may occur in cases where the marginal cost of diagnosis or interventions is very high and a judgment must be made on its effectiveness. Most rationing is justified on the grounds of scarcity or that no treatment in medicine can be said to offer an absolutely certain benefit for an individual patient. At the same time, this is also part of the controversy surrounding rationing because it is a question of judging whether the potential benefit can justify the expense. Rationing tends to have a negative connotation, implying tough decisions and restrictions. However, it is argued that if nations attempted to meet all healthcare needs, this would actually undermine the capacity to supply other basic needs or social goods such as public safety, education and defence because of lack of funding (Sheunemann & White, 2011).

Rationing thus brings into play the question of ethics because as the British Medical Association's Ethics Committee underlines: "Health professionals have an ethical duty to make the best use of the available resources and this means that hard decisions must be made" (BMA, 1999, p. 20, as quoted in Williams, 2001).

Rationing has become very central in the search for efficiency gains and to solve the funding crisis that the NHS is currently facing. Klein and Maybin (2012) identify several forms of rationing: rationing by denial, whereby commissioners refuse to fund particular treatments or establish lists for certain treatments that will not be funded by the NHS (such as surgery for lower back pain, cosmetic surgery, etc.), rationing by selection, where only certain patients can receive funding, rationing by deterrence, where patients are discouraged from using a service or applying for healthcare because of the various obstacles to access, rationing by deflection, whereby commissioners refuse spending and divert it to social services and, finally, rationing by dilution, whereby a service continues to be supplied but the quality declines due to staff cuts or obsolete equipment not being replaced. At the same time, rationing is also described as necessary to meet the rising costs of health systems. The development of NICE was seen as a way of making rationing fair because it became based on clinical and economic expertise. However, there is still scope for subjective rationing and unfair practices despite this framework. Governance plays an important part in rationing, or what policymakers refer to as priority setting. Decisions must be made on what services can be supplied, where funding should be allocated or reduced and cost-utility or cost-effectiveness analysis is used to maximise the impact of the input of resources. Resources must be allocated to produce the biggest increment in welfare and therefore must be the most cost-effective. A utilitarian approach is thus taken, but it is questionable whether this approach is really fair.

Klein and Maybin (2013) claim that the financial crisis has seen the rise of a distorted form of rationing: postcode rationing, rationing at a geographical level. For example, CCGs practice rationing which may cause disparities in supply. One example of this is the supply of In Vitro Fertilisation (IVF) treatment. Free IVF treatment has been restricted by NHS CCGs in some localities in recent years. While NICE make recommendations about who should have access to IVF treatment in England and Wales, individual CCGs make the final decision on who should have NHS-funded IVF in their catchment area. NICE recommends that women under 40 should be offered three cycles and women aged 40 to 42 one cycle if they have been trying to get pregnant for at least two years. However, some CCGs have extra criteria which may include not already having any children, being a healthy weight or not smoking. Some also lower the age range (for example to under 35 years) and only offer one cycle regardless of the age of the patient (NHS UK, 2020). A number of CCGs halted or suspended IVF treatment owing to financial restrictions in 2017. The NHS funded the lowest level of IVF cycles in England in 2017 (35%). The situation was better in Scotland (62%), in Northern Ireland (50%) and marginally better in Wales (39%) (HFEA, 2019). The Fertility Network UK's annual audit of CCGs in the UK, found that only 13% of all CCGs in England offered three full cycles of IVF in 2017. Seven CCGs offered no NHS IVF at all, and one in ten CCGs were looking to cut or remove NHS fertility treatment (Fertilitynetwork UK, 2018). This means that an increasing number of infertile couples have to fund IVF treatment themselves. The cost of private treatment varies. One cycle of IVG can cost £5000 or more and there may be additional costs for medicines, consultations and tests (NHS UK, 2020). IVF often exceeds £10,000 if all additional expenses are taken into account (NHS UK, 2020).

Rationing can have a significant impact on the provision of good quality healthcare. As Klein and Maybin (2012) underline, inefficiencies in the NHS are not always about lack of capacity or poor management, but more about strategic rationing. The authors give the example of longer waiting lists as a strategic complexity in the governance process. The cause of longer waiting lists is often due to the deferring of treatment to the next financial year. There is a maximum waiting time of 18 weeks, but commissioners will often push the waiting lists to their maximum.

But perhaps the most uneven form of rationing, similar to the IVF example and which obviously leads to uneven supply of health services, is 'bedside rationing'. 'Bedside rationing' can be described as "withholding by a physician of a medically beneficial service because of that service's cost to someone other than the patient" (Ubel & Goold, 1997, p. 75). Bedside rationing has three different forms: the physician (1) withholds, withdraws or fails to recommend a service that is in the patient's best medical interests; (2) acts to promote the financial interests of someone other than the patient and (3) controls the use of the medically beneficial service (Ubel & Goold, 1997).

Examples may include physicians as well as commissioners internalising resource constraints and reducing the number of drugs, MRI scans, etc. Bedside rationing is evident in many areas of health and particularly when budgets are very tight. However, there is another important means by which the NHS has tried to reduce costs to avoid rationing and that is by contracting out services to the private sector.

Increasing the Role of the Private Sector in Public Healthcare Delivery

With the introduction of market mechanisms within the NHS, outlined in the first chapter, there is a significant debate on the effects of introducing private investment into the publicly funded NHS. According to physician Jeoffry Gordon (2009), healthcare cannot be aligned with the market because it is not an ordinary commodity and is much closer to a public good. He defines a public good as a product or service which benefits everyone in the community. It requires large initial investment costs, which are too expensive for an individual to afford or for a private corporation to provide and keep afloat or make a reasonable return. Nevertheless, Gordon admits that health does have some characteristics that align it to the market and others that make it different from other goods. First, healthcare is not demanded because it is pleasurable but because the individual wishes to improve his or her health. The outcome is thus more important than the immediate pleasure. On the other hand, the good can be manufactured (if we think of x-rays), it is a product in demand for which people are willing to pay and it remains scarce relative to people's requirements. Thus, in this way, it cannot be considered entirely as a public good. Moreover, health is not just affected by healthcare but by other areas of welfare. However, health differs from other commodities in that the needs of the population essentially come before any other considerations.

Demand for healthcare can be linked to other goods and services, but it has specific features which mean that the usual resource allocation effects of the market are not applicable. The vast majority of health professionals, government officials and the population request that healthcare be provided on the basis of need, which means that a conventional market is unsuitable. As Marc Wuyts argues: "Public goods are socially defined and constructed according to what is perceived as a 'public need,' rather than containing certain inherent characteristics of non-excludability and non-rivalry (Wuyts, 2002, p. 30).

This does not mean to say that some actors of the health sector are not part of the market process, aligned with a competitive market: pharmaceutical companies, providers of services like dentistry, ophthalmic services and pharmaceutical dispensing all conform to the perfect or near perfect market model. However, others actors, such as hospitals, are aligned with public good requirements and needs-based criteria. As Royo-Bordonada and Román-Maestre (2015) underline, a public good or service invariably implies the involvement of governments to preserve the health of the population, which means that public health is inevitably paternalistic and utilitarian, because what matters is preserving the health of the maximum number of individuals.

Moreover, unlike with conventional goods, the patient is never really the consumer. Most purchasing decisions are not taken by the patient but by the doctor who acts as the patient's surrogate. The doctor who provides the care or recommends external care has little or no information about the patient's purchasing power. He does not take financial considerations into account because the patient may need urgent care very quickly and this will be his priority and is part and parcel of professional ethics. It is therefore very difficult to negotiate a price in such a configuration because healthcare services do not really belong to a conventional commercial marketplace and, when they are aligned to the market, it is still necessary to take into consideration non-market norms, notably values and institutions, whether they be governments or public interest entities.

Yet the process of audit, inspection and reviews and the growing need to be accountable and get value for money have reduced the scope of the public in health services. With particular reference to England's health system, Brown and Baker (2012) argue that neo-liberalism has led to a health service defined by non-collective, low-cost solutions to the problem of growing welfare budgets, deinstitutionalisation of healthcare, privatisation of services and the adoption of 'user pays' models. Financial austerity has thus led to a conception of health as a private responsibility and a move away from the welfarist view which held that the state was responsible for regulating and upholding both individual and collective wellbeing.

Financial considerations have also meant the principle of margin, i.e. the cost or benefit incurred with changing allocations of resources, is sometimes applied to public health, even if such analysis raises many difficulties. Public health systems must take into consideration the extra cost incurred by adding one additional unit of production, and if the marginal cost rises above the average cost health policymakers have to decide whether it is worthwhile providing such services. Efficiency also comes into play in current health systems. The mantra of governments over the last decades has indeed been to make the best use of scarce resources to deliver health to the population. Our health systems function more and more along a Pareto criterion: that is, providing a service which makes some people better off, but nobody worse off (i.e. a Pareto optimum). So, it would seem that Pareto efficiency or allocative efficiency is evident in health services, i.e. public authorities will take into consideration the appropriate allocation of resources in health that will be accepted by the population. An economic approach to managing the health system has thus replaced the old welfarist model. It may make sense economically, but also raises serious ethical and equity issues when it is the state which implements such policies since democratic states are supposed to be committed to treating all citizens in the same way.

The ethics argument is often used by critics against introducing market forms of governance in the health service. Such critics argue that the values upon which the NHS were founded and market forces are incompatible because healthcare shows that there is a moral limit to markets. Given that health is dependent on value judgments, the ethic perspective relating to health cannot be ignored. In philosophy, ethics can be defined as a critical rational reflection on morals. However, in health it refers to the field of study and practice of understanding the values guiding decisions and actions in healthcare, health research and health policy. It encompasses much more than medical ethics, which is looking at ethical issues within the clinical areas and bioethics, and relates to the health of all living things. Health ethics includes all kinds of decision making in clinical care, health services and systems and public health overall. Public health ethics incorporates equity, solidarity, social justice, reciprocity and trust. Public health ethics also implies collective action to protect health.

It can be argued that processes may be unethical and therefore cannot be used even if they help to improve the health of the population. Some ethical theories are directed at institutions and how they might achieve greater social justice. Yet ethics are difficult to describe and pin down because the concept is not descriptive but normative and amounts to deciding which morals are legitimate (Limentani, 1999). The very understanding of public health is dependent on the ethical perspective taken. Limentani (1999) underlines that decisions for health are therefore justified according to moral decisions and actions. Present day healthcare presents different moral difficulties because of the multidisciplinary actors involved in healthcare delivery, including managers, boards and governments.

Some would argue that there is a role for the private sector in all areas of public healthcare provision. Indeed, the US Institute of Medicine (IOM) (2003) contends that public health can be delivered by both public and private organisations and agencies because public health depends on what society and its agents are capable of doing to ensure that people are healthy. Nevertheless, it is important not to underestimate Kenneth Arrow's analysis of the lack of information in public services, which raise difficulties for the provision of healthcare by private suppliers:

The value of information is frequently not known in any meaningful sense to the buyer; if, indeed, he knew enough to measure the value of information, he would know the information itself. But information in the form of skilled care is precisely what is being bought from most physicians, and, indeed, from most professionals. The elusive character of information as a commodity suggests that it departs considerably from the usual marketability assumptions about commodities (Arrow, 1963, p.18).

So such information asymmetries result in serious inefficiencies in private purchasing and pricing, because individuals are sometimes unable to assess whether they need medical treatment and, especially, when and what kind of treatment they need. The same applies to private insurers, which makes risk-analysis tricky.

The privatisation of the NHS, or more accurately the marketisation of the NHS, is thus a very controversial subject because of the arguments in favour of maintaining public health as a public good. Detractors are also concerned about the negative impacts of competition and profit for patient services, finances and health ethics. In the conclusion of their publication, Rothgang (2010) defines three forms of privatisation that have taken place in the British health system following the Griffiths reform of 1984 described in the previous chapter. First, functional privatisation, which has involved the outsourcing of hospital catering and cleaning to private providers. Second, material privatisation, which is the provision of hospital beds by private and international providers, dental and long-term care private providers. In addition, consultants have increased their provision of private services using NHS facilities. Finally, formal privatisation with directly managed units being transformed into independent NHS trust hospitals.

Successive governments since the late 1980s (both left and right) have gradually put in place a system which allows private providers to compete with each other to offer services to the NHS. New Labour extended the use of

Private Finance Iniatives (PFIs) in the NHS, creating NHS Local Improvement Finance Trusts (LIFTs). In 2008, 48 NHS LIFTs had been contracted along with other Private Finance Initiatives (PFIs). Private Finance Initiatives (PFIs) contracted for the building of hospitals have nevertheless been criticised. While contractors argue that the PFIs enable projects to be completed more quickly, critics argue that PFIs are more expensive. PFI locks the NHS into long-term contracts and providers often need to be supported by other sources of finance to cover the full costs (Pollock, 2004; Ham, 2009).

The extension of the Private Finance Initiative in the health sector has also been heavily criticised by both the popular and the quality press. Services outsourced to private companies through PFI led to the compulsory redundancies of 4,620 frontline NHS staff between 2010/11 and 2012/13, and 2,430 voluntary redundancies. Since 2010, more than 30 NHS maternity and 42 A&E units have either been closed down or downgraded. Until 1990, hospitals did not have to pay a charge for their land, building and assets, but PFI hospitals must pay more than 15% of annual operating costs. Since the launching of the PFI in 1992, there has been an association with trust mergers which has led to a 30% reduction of hospital beds, staff lay-offs and closures of hospitals and community services (Campbell, 2013). The hospitals are closed down because the government does not allow PFI hospitals to default on debt to avoid threatening other PFI schemes. Such negative impacts can explain the criticism of the aforementioned contracts.

PFIs have more recently come into the public light with the collapse of Carillon[1] which had contracted a number of PFIs with NHS hospitals. Vital construction of two hospitals thus came to a halt in mid-January 2018. A significant outlay had been made to Carillon to build the £335 million Royal Liverpool University hospital in Mersyside and the £350 million Midland Metropolitan hospital in Smethwick. Such projects had proved to have a significant underestimated outlay for the company. Companies that take on PFI projects are actually operating on very small profit margins or to a loss if the projects are beset by problems. However, private companies are willing to take on such construction deals because they are given a large bulk sum of cash up front, which can be used to pay off other debts. Such was the case with Carillon (Goodley, 2018). As a result, Theresa May's government declared in the 2018 Autumn Budget Statement that no more PFIs would be contracted.

In addition, under New Labour, in an attempt to reduce patient waiting lists and hit targets, Independent Sector Treatment Centres (ISTCs) were created. A number of private Canadian and South African companies provide care in ISTCs offering general and specialist surgery services. Partnerships have also been set up between US-based healthcare companies and the NHS. However, very little research has been carried out on ISTCs because of a lack of published contract data and poor quality data returns (Pollock & Kirkwood, 2009). One study published in 2011 suggested that ISTCs provided "at least as good" care as that provided by the NHS (Bardsley, 2011).

Barnabas, Clarke, & Leaver (2014) argue that there may be some room for market methods in health services but the competition mantra on which the Health and Social Care Act of 2012 is founded goes too far from an economic and moral stance. Indeed, the Health and Social Care Act which came into force on 1 April 2013 has increased the implication of the private sector. As Matthews argues:

The decisive factor, as in other sectors of the welfare state, has been the neoliberal push to remake healthcare in the image of the "free market." In England, the greatest single blow to universal healthcare in the NHS's history came with the enactment of the Health and Social Care Act (HSCA) in 2012 (Matthews, 2017, para. 19).

He goes on to explain how the law actually abolished the NHS's founding principles of guaranteeing universal care because the Secretary of State is no longer responsible for the promotion in England of a comprehensive health service. The government is still responsible for funding healthcare, however the direct responsibility for providing healthcare to its citizens is that of the autonomous body Healthcare England. It is estimated that in the year following the enforcement of this Act, £13 billion in NHS contracts was advertised, which is almost three times greater than the previous year and a 30% increase in advertising, encouraging bids from private groups and charities and representing over 70 different services, compared to 40 in 2012. Matthews (2017) also argues that £200 million in contracts was also made with business services and the consulting industry, to firms such as Ernst and Young, Deloitte and McKinsey.

Moreover, under the terms of the Health and Social Care Act of 2012, trusts can earn up to 49% of their total income from private services. In addition, it has granted CCGs 'real' budgets to buy care on behalf of their local communities, which has encouraged more tendering to the private sector because CCGs control about £60 billion of the NHS budget and are responsible for commissioning local services. Therefore, extra focus is actually put on commissioning. Commissioning takes place through competitive tendering and NHS contracts are therefore open for tender to the voluntary and private sectors. This has led to £250 million worth of NHS services being put out to tender, with 105 private firms granted contracts (Watt, 2014).

The reconfiguration of the NHS and the implementation of recent health legislation have also encouraged NHS consultants to increasingly engage in private activity. Although specialist consultants have always had the right to practice alongside their NHS work, it was nevertheless limited until 1980. Full-time NHS consultants did not have the right to provide private healthcare. Part-time NHS consultants were allowed to practice without restrictions, but had to accept a reduction in their salary (Webster, 2002). However, the conservative governments of the 1980s gradually reduced these restrictions, allowing both full and part-time consultants to conduct private consultations without any salary reduction, although full-time consultants were only allowed to earn up to 10% of their income from private work. The Health and Social Care Act of 2012 has now removed all caps on private earnings.

Since its enactment, this law has been heavily criticised, particularly section 75 which obliges commissioners to make calls for tenders for all services. Private contractors are now more likely than public constractors to win these tenders. This regulation acts, in this way, as the driving force behind the privatisation of the NHS, giving private companies the opportunity to provide NHS services where they are likely to make the most profit. Companies such as Care UK or Virgin Care tend to bid for the most profitable services - diagnostics, elective surgery and simple treatments, for example - leaving responsibility for emergency medical care, elderly care, mental health services and anything else that is not necessarily profitable to the public market. According to the UK Department of Health and Social Care 2019 annual report, a record number of contracts were awarded to the private sector, totaling £9.2 billion for the period 2018/9 (Department of Health and Social Care, 2019). Virgin Care has contracts worth hundreds of millions of pounds, running more than 230 NHS and social care services. Other private companies that have shown an active interest to take on NHS services are Bio Product Laboratories (BPL), Care UK, Circle, General Healthcare Group (GHG), HCA International (Hospital Corporation of America), Ramsay, Spire Healthcare, The Practice PLC and United Health (Optum). International operators are numerous in the provision of hospital beds such as General Healthcare Group, a US for-profit hospital provider (see Table 1).

In March 2018, a survey of the state of privatisation of healthcare in Britain was carried out by the Centre for Health and the Public Interest (Walpole, 2018). It found that the total income that the NHS had generated from private patients had increased by 16% over the four years since the enactment of the

Table 1. Private provider summaries

GP / Community Care	
Virgin Care	One of the leading private providers in the NHS. Active in primary care and community services. Provides over 400 services to the NHS according to the company website in mid-2017, including GP services, urgent care, musculoskeletal, sexual health, integrated children's services. The company has targeted some large contracts and since 2010 has been awarded contracts worth over £2.5 billion by NHS organisations.
Care UK	Day care and homes for the elderly. GP services, diagnostics, Community Assessment and Treatment Services (CATS), treatment centres, mental health services, eating disorder services, learning disability services. Receives income from the NHS of over £350 million per year.
The Practice	Provider of primary care services and delivers specialist clinical services to GPs. Network of surgeries. Acquired United Health Primary Care in 2011 from United Health UK – six practices. The US company Centene owns 75% of the company.
United Health/ Optum	Wide range of services for NHS – Health Needs assessment, GP Commissioning, clinical services redesign, performance & contract management, Care solutions, Medicines management. No longer involved with GP practices.
Serco	Range of non-clinical services, including prisons, facilities management, IT and payroll services. Exited the clinical market in 2015 after a number of problems.
Nestor Primecare	Home care, care homes, mental health services, children's services, out-of-hours, dentistry and primary care (as Primecare).
Totally plc	This company is active in the area of out of hospital care, including physiotherapy, podiatry, dermatology, Referral Management Services and Clinical Health Coaching. The company has built up its business through acquisitions, including in Premier Physical Healthcare Ltd, About Health Ltd in 2016 and in October 2017, Vocare Ltd; the latter company added urgent care and out-of-hours services. The company is listed on the AIM market of the London Stock Exchange.
Hospitals	
Circle	Private hospitals: Circle Bath, Circle Reading; clinics: Windsor, Nottingham. Pulled out of ten-year contract to run Hinchingbrooke hospital early 2015 after only two years. Circle is now targeting large community care contracts and in 2014 won a contract to run musculoskeletal services in Bedfordshire.
General Healthcare (BMI, Netcare)	Owned by General Healthcare with over 70 facilities UK-wide. GHG also consists of Care Fertility, a private specialist in fertility treatment, and Netcare, a network of clinics set up in 2002 in the UK by South African company Netcare, which undertakes work under contract to the NHS.
Spire / Classic	Second largest private healthcare hospital group in the UK with 37 hospitals. The major part of Spire's business (61% in 2010) is from the private medical insurance market, but NHS admissions accounted for 25% of its business in 2010, followed by 14% from self-paying customers.
HCA International	HCA International is one of the smaller private hospital groups in the UK, with a network of only six hospitals and four outpatient clinics, all in the London area. Partnerships with leading NHS hospital trusts.
Ramsay (plus Capio)	Ramsay Health UK has a network of 22 acute hospitals in the UK delivering both private treatment and care under contract to the NHS.
Mental Health Services	
Partnerships in Care	Largest independent provider of secure mental health facilities across the UK.
Priory Group	Provider of acute mental healthcare, secure and step down services, specialist education, complex care and neuro-rehabilitation services, fostering and care homes.

continues on following page

Table 1. Continued

Diagnostics	
Alliance (Lodestone)	Diagnostics for the NHS and independent sector.
InHealth Group Ltd	InHealth provide diagnostics for NHS patients throughout the UK and Ireland.
IT/Support Services/Commissioning	
Capita	IT, patient engagement, HR, payroll, estates, commissioning services
Centene	IT, digital technologies
CapGemini	IT
McKesson	IT
Mouchel	Commissioning services
BDO	Commissioning services
Interserve	Support services

Source: NHS Support Federation, 2018

Health and Social Care Act of 2012. The main concern about privatisation that emerged from the survey was that 1% of NHS's 131,000 beds were occupied or put aside for private patients. This may appear small, however the number of NHS beds is constantly falling and total occupancy rates at dangerous levels (95% or more in winter months), which represents a significant loss for the treatment of NHS-funded patients (Ewbank et al. 2018, Walpole, 2018).

Yet the increased involvement of the private sector in the provision of public health services brings with it significant administrative costs. In 2010, the Health Select Committee reported that the cost of running the NHS as a market took up 14% of the NHS budget each year. The same committee pointed out that in the period before the market was introduced in the NHS, in the late 1980s, administration only accounted for 5% of the NHS budget (National Health Action Party, 2015). Even though the administration costs might have risen anyway as a proportion of the budget, it would seem that the marketisation of public health services does tend to have more transaction costs – advertising, negotiating contracting, invoicing, billing, auditing, monitoring contracts, collecting information, resolving disputes both in court and out, etc. NHS providers have also been criticised for the pay of their Chief Executives and hiring expensive management consultants. The CCGs are advised by costly Commissioning Support Units (CSUs), which were created under the Coalition government. Regulation to ensure the fair play of the market sector also costs money, which is overseen by the NHS Trust Development Authority Monitor and the Care Quality Commission (CQC) among other entities, etc. (National Health Action Party, 2015).

Removing these costs could free up funds to make up for the NHS shortfall and provide critical social care if market activities were reduced. A comparison with Scotland's hospital administration costs shows that in a less marketised system, there are fewer transaction costs. In the USA where one healthcare dollar in every three is spent on administration because of a significantly privatised system, international score boards reveal poorer outcomes than in the NHS (OECD, 2017).

There are also a number of other concerns over introducing private markets in healthcare. As Nobel Laureate Kenneth Arrow stated in 1963 "patients are not customers in a supermarket" (quoted in Thomas, 2015). It takes expertise that the common patient simply does not have and therefore choice should not be an issue. A marketised system also tends to provide incentives to overtreat, overinvestigate and stimulate patient demand through advertising. There is also evidence that marketisation in the NHS has compromised care. In the Francis report that examined the failures of care at Mid Staffordshire[2], it was found that too much emphasis had been put on the market in running the hospital in order to get Foundation Trust status, which ended up compromising co-operation between medical professionals (Francis, 2013). Hinchinbrooke hospital, which is more or less run through the private sector, was also criticised by the Royal College of Surgeons and the CQC for poor standards of care and demoralised staff (BBC, 2012).

NHS Chief Executive Simon Stevens has argued for an end to the NHS market structure, which currently gives separate roles to purchasers and providers. Stevens said the system should be replaced by integration of services and joint planning between different providers. This Act goes further than the conservative reforms of the 1980s, as it uses the purchaser-provider division, not only as it once did as a means of managing the service, but for the functioning of the entire system of care (Timmins, 2018). As a result, one of the greatest risks is the expansion of private healthcare (nationally and internationally) and a crowding out effect on public health sector investment. This means that the best doctors and/or health specialists may then decide to turn to the private sector as well as wealthier citizens, leaving a less efficient public health system for the poorest. The move towards a market system and reliance on private providers thus remains controversial.

CONCLUSION

Financial governance has become an important part of public health service delivery in the UK. Increased funding pressures means that there are more financial controls and healthcare providers must justify financial outlays. Introducing fees for service users or alternative forms of income to meet costs have been ruled out because they are too problematic and costly to roll out. However, contracting out and welcoming of private patients within the NHS have been ways in which health service providers have attempted to reduce service costs with mixed results. Yet one of the biggest costs for the NHS is staff (see Figure 3), which is also the most difficult overhead to reduce. Any drive in the past to cut costs has led to a decline in morale and departures leading to staff shortages, a question which will be examined in more detail in the next chapter.

Figure 3. Breakdown of Clinical Commissioning Groups' total expenditure, 2017-18
Source: NAO (2018)

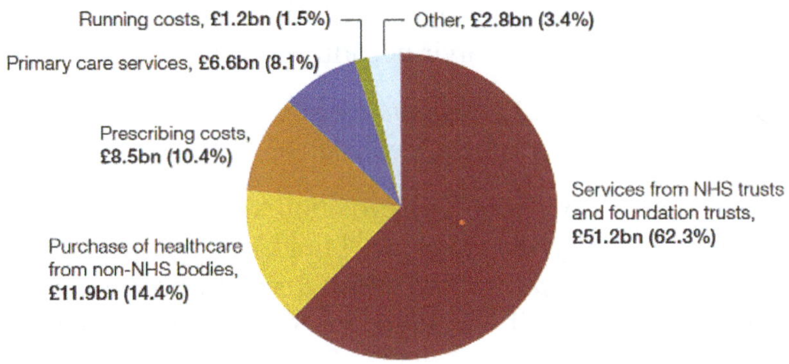

REFERENCES

Arrow, K. J. (1963). Uncertainty and the welfare economics of medical care. *The American Economic Review*, *53*(5), 941–973.

Bardsley, M., & Dixon, J. (2011, November 4). Quality of care in Independent Sector Treatment Centres. *BMJ (Clinical Research Ed.)*, *343*(nov04 1), d6936. doi:10.1136/bmj.d6936 PMID:22058122

Barker, K. (2014). *A new settlement for health and social care: Final report*. The King's Fund.

Barnabas, J. G., Clarke, E., & Leaver, L. (2014). Morality and markets in the NHS. *International Journal of Health Policy and Management*, *3*(7), 371–376. doi:10.15171/ijhpm.2014.123 PMID:25489594

BBC News. (2012, March 7). *Hinchingbrooke hospital 'sorry' for bowel cancer shortcomings*. Retrieved March 8, 2019, from https://www.bbc.com/news/uk-england-cambridgeshire-17285379

Boseley, S. (2015, January 16). Hepatitis C drug delayed by NHS due to high cost. *The Guardian*. Retrieved January 8, 2018, from https://www.theguardian.com/society/2015/jan/16/sofosbuvir-hepatitis-c-drug-nhs

Brown, B., & Baker, S. (2012). *Responsible citizens: Individuals, health and policy under neoliberalism*. Anthem Press. doi:10.7135/UPO9780857289131

Camp-Pietrain, E. (2019, September). Devolution and health policy in Scotland: A model for sustainability and efficiency? In L. Dalingwater (Ed.), *Seventy years on: Framing health policy in Britain, Revue française de civilisation britannique*. Retrieved April 10, 2020, from https://journals.openedition.org/rfcb/4105

Campbell, D. (2013, December 21). 7,000 key NHS clinical staff made redundant amid enforced cuts. *The Guardian*. Retrieved December 6, 2018, from <www.theguardian.com/society/2013/dec/31/nhs-staff-laid-offamid-savings-drive

Campbell, D. (2015, May 6). NHS "like sick patient in early-stage terminal decline", former boss says. *The Guardian*. Retrieved September 3, 2017, from https://www.theguardian.com/society/2015/may/06/nhs-like-sick-patient-in-early-stage-terminal-decline-former-boss-says

Claxton, K. (2007). OFT, VBP: QED? *Health Economics*, *16*(6), 545–558. doi:10.1002/hec.1249 PMID:17535009

Cockburn, H. (2017, 30 December). NHS privatisation soars as private companies win 70% of clinical contracts in England. *Independent*. Retrieved June 10, 2018, from https://www.independent.co.uk/news/health/nhs-privatisation-contracts-virgin-care-richard-branson-jeremy-hunt-a8134386.html

Department of Health and Social Care. (2019, May 24). *Speech delivered by Matt Hancock: Better tech will build better relationships between clinicians and patients*. Retrieved April 6, 2020, from https://www.gov.uk/government/speeches/better-tech-will-build-better-relationships-between-clinicians-and-patients

Department of Health, Association of the British Pharmaceutical Industry. (2013). *Pharmaceutical price regulation scheme 2014*. Department of Health. Retrieved June 4, 2019, from www.gov.ukgovernment/publications/pharmaceutical-price-regulation-scheme-2014

Ewbank, L., Omojomolo, D., Sullivan, K., & McKenna, H. (2018, April). *The rising cost of medicines to the NHS. What's the story?* The King's Fund. Retrieved December 8, 2019, from: https://www.kingsfund.org.uk/sites/default/files/2018-04/Rising-cost-of-medicines.pdf

Fertilitynetwork, U. K. (2018). *Fertility Fairness Audit*. Retrieved April 10, 2020, from https://fertilitynetworkuk.org/fertility-fairness-audit/

Francis, R. (2013). *Report of the Mid-Staffordshire NHS Foundation Trust Public Inquiry*. Stationery Office. HC 947.

Goodley, S. (2018, January 15). The four contracts that finished Carillion. *The Guardian*. Retrieved January 5, 2019, from https://www.theguardian.com/business/2018/jan/15/the-four-contracts-that-finished-carillion-public-private-partnership

Gordon, J. B. (2009). Is healthcare a public good? *Physician Blog*. Retrieved September 6, 2017, from www.kevinmd.com/blog/2009/08/is-health-care-a-public-good.html

Ham, C. (2009). *Health policy in Britain* (6th ed.). Palgrave Macmillan. doi:10.1007/978-1-137-01397-2

Harker, R. (2020, January 17). *NHS expenditure*. House of Commons Library. Retrived on April 9, 2020, from https://commonslibrary.parliament.uk/research-briefings/sn00724/

Heginbotham, C. (1997). Why rationing is inevitable in the NHS. In B. New (Ed.), *Rationing: Talk and action in healthcare* (pp. 43–57). BMJ Publishing Group.

Human Fertilisation and Embryology Authority (HFEA). (2019). *Fertility treatment 2017: Trends and figures*. Retrieved April 10, 2020, from https://www.hfea.gov.uk/media/2894/fertility-treatment-2017-trends-and-figures-may-2019.pdf

Institute of Medicine (IOM). (2003). *The future of the public's health in the 21st Century*. The National Academies Press.

Klein, R., & Maybin, J. (2012). *Thinking about rationing*. The King's Fund.

Kollewe, J. (2017, November 21). Drug firm Concordia overcharged NHS with 6,000% price rise, says watchdog. *The Guardian*. Retrieved on September 3, 2018, from https://www.theguardian.com/business/2017/nov/21/drug-firm-concordia-overcharged-nhs-with-6000-price-rise

Komaromy, C. (2001). Caring for life: dilemmas in healthcare. In C. Komaromy (Ed.), *Dilemmas in UK healthcare* (pp. 11–20). Open University Press.

Lenaghan, J. (1997). Responses to the rationing agenda in the NHS. In B. New (Ed.), *Rationing: talk and action in healthcare* (pp. 31–40). BMJ Publishing Group.

Matthews, D. (2017, March). The battle for the National Health Service: England, Wales and the socialist vision. *Monthly Review*, *68*(10), 25. Retrived on November 4, 2018, from https://www.researchgate.net/publication/314206672_The_Battle_for_the_National_Health_Service_England_Wales_and_the_Socialist_Vision

McCarthney, M. (2015, July 20-26). Partnerships: pharma is closer than you think. *BMJ*, 351. 10.1136/bmj.h3688

Morgan-Bentley, P. (2018, February 2). NHS forced to pay £1,500 for £2 pot of moisturizer. *Financial Times*. Retrieved March 3, 2019, from https://www.thetimes.co.uk/article/nhs-forced-to-pay-1-500-for-2-pot-of-moisturiser-3d0ckn3gh

National Audit Office (NAO). (2018, December 18). *A review of the role and costs of clinical commissioning groups*. NAO. Retrieved April 12, 2020, from https://www.nao.org.uk/wp-content/uploads/2018/12/A-review-of-the-role-and-costs-of-clinical-commissioning-groups-Summary.pdf

National Health Action Party. (2015). *NHA's key pillars for a healthy NHS and a healthy population*. Retrieved February 13, 2017, from www.nhap.org

New, B. (1997). The rationing agenda in the NHS. In B. New (Ed.), *Rationing: Talk and action in healthcare* (pp. 8–30). BMJ Publishing Group.

NHS Digital. (2017). *Prescription cost analysis, England – 2016: data trends*. NHS Digital. Retrieved March 3, 2019, from https://digital.nhs.uk/catalogue/PUB23631

NHS England. (2014). *Memorandum of Understanding between NHS England, the Association of the British Pharmaceutical Industry (ABPI) and the British Generic Manufacturers Association (BGMA)*. NHS England. Retrieved November 8, 2019, from https://www.england.nhs.uk/wp-content/uploads/2014/10/memo-underst-25-09-14.pdf

NHS England. (2016). *Consolidated 2015/16 year-end financial report. Board paper for meeting on 26 May 2016, agenda item no. 7*. NHS England. Retrieved February 3, 2018, from www.england.nhs.uk/2016/05/board-meet-26-may-16/

NHS Information Centre. (2007). *Prescriptions dispensed in the community: Statistics for 1996 to 2006: England*. NHS Information Centre. Retrieved on August 2, 2017, from https://digital.nhs.uk/catalogue/PUB01318

NHS UK. (2020). *IVF*. Retrieved on April 10, 2020, from https://www.nhs.uk/conditions/ivf/availability/

OECD. (2017). *Health at a glance*. OECD.

OECD. (2019). *Health at a glance*. OECD.

ONS. (2018, August 13). *Living longer: How our population is changing and why it matters*. Retrieved February 4, 2019, from https://www.ons.gov.uk/peoplepopulationandcommunity/birthsdeathsandmarriages/ageing/articles/livinglongerhowourpopulationischangingandwhyitmatters/2018-08-13

Pollock, A. M. (2004). *NHS plc: The privatisation of our healthcare*. Verso.

Poole, T. (2008). *Briefing: NICE technology appraisals*. The King's Fund. Retrieved September 6, 2018, from www.kingsfund.org.uk/publications/nice-technology-appraisals

Rothgang, H. (2010). The converging role of the state in OECD healthcare systems. In H. Rothgang, M. Cacace, L. Frisina, S. Grimmeisen, A. Schmid, & C. Wendt (Eds.), *The state and healthcare: Comparing OECD countries* (pp. 237–247). Palgrave Macmillan. doi:10.1057/9780230292345_8

Royo-Bordonada, M. A., & Román-Maestre, B. (2015). Towards public health ethics. *Public Health Reviews*, *36*(3). Retrieved November 6, 2018, from publichealthreviews.biomedcentral.com/articles/10.1186/s40985-015-0005-0 PMID:29450031

Sheunemann, L., & White, D. (2011, December). The ethics and reality of rationing in medicine. *Chest*, *140*(6), 1625–1632. doi:10.1378/chest.11-0622 PMID:22147821

The Health Foundation. (2015, March). *Swimming against the tide? The quality of NHS services during the current parliament*. Briefing. Retrieved November 6, 2018, from www.health.org.uk/quality overview.

The King's Fund. (2015). *General Election 2015: Analysis*. King's Fund. Retrieved September 8, 2018, from www.kingsfund.org.uk/topics/general-election-2015

The King's Fund. (2017, November 7). *The Autumn Budget: Joint statement on health and social care*. Retrieved November 7, 2018, from https://www.kingsfund.org.uk/publications/autumn-budget-2017

The King's Fund. (2020, March 13). *The NHS budget and how it has changed*. Retrieved April 8, 2020, from https://www.kingsfund.org.uk/projects/nhs-in-a-nutshell/nhs-budget

Thomas, K. (2015, March 10). What the healthcare sector wants from the next government. *The Guardian*. Retrieved November 7, 2018, from https://www.theguardian.com/healthcare-network/2015/mar/10/healthcare-sector-wants-next-government

Timmins, N. (2017). *Ministers, not NHS England, should decide on the affordability of cost effective new treatments*. The King's Fund. Retrieved November 9, 2019, from www.kingsfund.org.uk/publications/articles/ministers-not-nhs-england-should-decide-affordability-of-treatments

Timmins, N. (2018, October 25). *Amending the 2012 Act: Can it be done*? King's Fund. Retrieved April 10, 2020, from https://www.kingsfund.org.uk/publications/amending-2012-act-can-it-be-done?utm_source=The%20King%27s%20Fund%20newsletters%20%28main%20account%29&utm_medium=email&utm_campaign=9951752_NEWSL_ICB%202018-11-14&dm_i=21A8%2C5XATK%2CFLWSXD%2CN6UID%2C1#the-legislative-outlook

Treasury, H. M. (2015). *Spending review 2015*. HM Treasury.

Ubel, P. A., & Goold, S. (1997). Recognizing bedside rationing: Clear cases and tough calls. *Annals of Internal Medicine*, *126*(1), 74–80. doi:10.7326/0003-4819-126-1-199701010-00010 PMID:8992926

Walpole, S. (2018, March). *NHS treatment of private patients*. CHPI. Retrieved on November 8, 2019, from https://chpi.org.uk/wp-content/uploads/2018/03/CHPI-NHS-Private-Patients-Mar18.pdf

Watt, N. (2014, August 19). Income from private patients soars at NHS hospital trusts. *The Guardian*. Retrieved September 8, 2017, from https://www.theguardian.com/society/2014/aug/19/private-patient-income-soars-nhs-privatisation

Webster, C. (2002). *The National Health Service – A political history*. Oxford University Press.

Williams, A. (2001). Dilemmas in healthcare: Responding to economic constraints. In C. Komaromy (Ed.), *Dilemmas in UK healthcare* (pp. 21–39). Open University Press.

Wuyts, M. (2002). Deprivation and public need. In M. Macintosh & M. Wuyts (Eds.), *Development policy and public action* (pp. 13–37). Oxford University Press.

ENDNOTES

1 Carillon plc. was a British construction and services company with headquarters in Wolverhampton. After experiencing financial difficulties in 2017, it went into compulsory liquidation on 15 January 2018.

2 The Mid Staffordshire failure of care, which led to an enquiry, involved two hospitals in Mid Staffordshire where hundreds of hospital patients died as a result of sub-standard care and staff failings between January 2005 and March 2009. Investigations showed that patients lay in wards starving, thirsty and in soiled bedclothes. Other patients received the wrong medication or none at all. Receptionists were taking decisions about which patients should be treated and nurses were reported to be incapable of using equipment and were therefore switching it off.

Chapter 3
The Role of Health Professionals

ABSTRACT

Staff governance is a major challenge for the NHS. It refers to the framework for managing employees in the National Health Service (NHS). Professional practitioners, in particular doctors and nurses, have a key role to play in the running of the NHS, but there are many challenges in managing staff and especially ensuring high retention levels. This chapter begins by explaining the power relations within the NHS and among some of the key actors. It then highlights some of the key challenges including those posed by the loss of European Union (EU) staff following the UK's decision to leave the EU. In particular, it explains why it has become increasingly difficult in recent years to retain staff in the NHS. It then discusses some of the measures to stem the haemorrhaging of staff.

INTRODUCTION

While the move from public administration forms of governance to New Public Management (NPM) has diminished the influence of professional practitioners, especially in England, doctors and nurses do still have a key role to play in the running of public health services and can influence policymaking. Alford underlines the key role that professionals play in health politics governed by a combination of 'professional monopolists' (i.e. health professionals) who represent the dominion interests, 'corporate rationalisers' (executive

DOI: 10.4018/978-1-7998-3928-6.ch003

managers from the private sector) who may challenge those interests and the 'community population' (patients) who may repress these interests (Alford, 1975). Although the drafting in of managers from the private sector may have altered the nature of governance, it has not necessarily reduced the influence of doctors and medical professionals (Ham, 2009). Indeed, Ham argues that the decline of corporatist governance may have weakened doctors' power in influencing national policy but they still have significant influence at the micro-level. This chapter will thus consider the role of professionals in the governance framework. It will then examine some of the main workforce challenges of the National Health Service (NHS), namely staff shortages and future departures following Britain's vote to leave the European Union (EU).

POWER RELATIONS AND FRONTLINE STAFF

The medical profession is represented at all levels of decision making in the NHS. For example, in the Department of Health, the Chief Medical Officer and NHS Medical Director are senior doctors. National clinical directors from this professional corpus are also present in the department to lead policy on clinical priorities such as cancer and coronary heart disease (Ham, 2009). In the Clinical Commissioning Groups (CCGs), which now govern the administration of health services at the local level in England, many of the senior managers have a medical background (for example many of the clinical leads and other CCG managers are senior nurses). The principles of resource management are based on involving senior practitioners in the management of hospitals and primary care, inherited from the clinical governance framework set up by New Labour.

According to historian Rudolf Klein, the creation of the NHS in 1948 was not necessarily welcomed by doctors. He underlines that the NHS has continued to have a power struggle ever since of 'keeping the doctors happy' while still making them accountable and adhering to reforms and governance principles (Klein, 2013). Politicians and health managers continually struggle to push through reforms because of the influence of doctors and nurses resisting them. The essential governance struggle between politicians, administrators and clinical practitioners has been over the latter arguing that the former two do not understand clinical needs, and therefore any political actions regarding the NHS will have unforeseen results. Since its conception, doctors have seen a move from complete independence, before the creation of the National Health Service, to semi-independence in the early days when doctors 'just got on with their work' and 'didn't have to report to anybody' to the situation today where managers from outside have altered the nature of the power and leeway of doctors and nurses. This is particularly the case in England which has seen a move towards market governance.

According to Dayan and Edwards (2017), Scotland has quite a different governance framework in place whereby the relations between the professionals on the frontline, government and different tiers of hierarchy are closer and less formal[1]. Scotland's public health system does not rely on hard incentives, process or access indicators, but rather patient outcomes. There are fewer tiers of hierarchy in Scotland than in England. Board chief executives have closer relations and meet more regularly with central civil servants and ministers. This contrasts with the more formal command and control system in England with inter-personal distance between front line staff, managers and government officials, and more tiers of hierarchy. Dayan and Edwards (2017) argue that the Scottish system inspires trust among frontline staff, working through persuasion rather than incentives. Policies for improvement and change tend to be devised and implemented by frontline professionals and rolled out across the board if successful. In contrast, in England, most pilot schemes are designed at the centre (by the government or NHS England) and then implemented. Managers drafted in from the private sector claim that clinical practitioners are strongly involved in the governance process, but that some refuse to engage in it. This might well be because of the lack of consultation in all key processes of design and the aforementioned difficulties to inspire trust in a more market-oriented and hierarchical system.

But, even in England, the essential role that doctors and nurses play in the health and wellbeing of the population means that if the professionals are unhappy with decisions, they can hold the government to ransom by threatening to resign *en masse*. For example, Margaret Thatcher managed to bring both public and private workers under her control. However, she struggled in her attempts to do the same to the doctors when changes to General Practitioners (GPs)' budgets were proposed under her premiership, although the reforms were eventually pushed through and extended under New Labour (Klein, 2013). Significant protests still take place such as that of the 2016 junior doctors' dispute in England, which was over the proposed modification to their contracts. Basic pay was to be increased by 13.5% on average, but changes to other parts of their pay package, such as guaranteed pay increase linked to seniority and the terms of 'unsociable hours' such as weekends, caused significant unrest. Thousands of operations were cancelled during the dispute (BBC, 2016). The safety issue means that doctors do have the power to hold the nation to ransom to a certain extent, although their professional ethics prevent them from doing this on a regular basis.

Globalisation has also meant that young doctors can actually train in Britain and then leave to get better pay in other countries such as Australia. The global marketplace means that if doctors are not happy with conditions in Britain, they will go elsewhere. The government and health service managers have difficulty in exerting control over senior doctors because they make decisions about the health organisation's resources and what happens to patients and they also have significant clinical authority. Doctors have substantial support as a group, financial independence and high salaries and the possibility to choose from public, private or international practices. Managers cannot therefore take a top-down approach and must negotiate to achieve targets in order to avoid strikes or disruption, which could lead to operation cancellations and significant health risks (Cox, 2001).

In England, in some ways, power has been given back to the professionals, particularly since the introduction of clinical governance. GPs, but also senior nurses in CCGs, are responsible for managing the administration because they are seen to be the most knowledgeable about how innovative practices can be introduced into the health sector. In practice, however, this has simply meant switching accountability to the professionals, who have become directly responsible for achieving the performance targets set out by the government and governmental agencies. Indeed, a BMA survey carried out in 2013 showed that in practice doctors were unable to push through changes to improve services because of lack of capacity (funding and support) (BMA, 2013). They also have to answer to standards set by individual patients because of the bigger role individuals have been granted through legislation to become involved in healthcare, such as the Care Act of 2014. Doctors and nurses are thus constantly challenged in this complex framework of decision making which involves not only the government but administrators, local services and the general public to whom they stand accountable. Yet one of the biggest governance challenges for the NHS at large is to retain qualified frontline staff and this is a challenge across the four nations of the UK.

Figure 1. Career Framework for the NHS
Source: NHS Careers (2020)

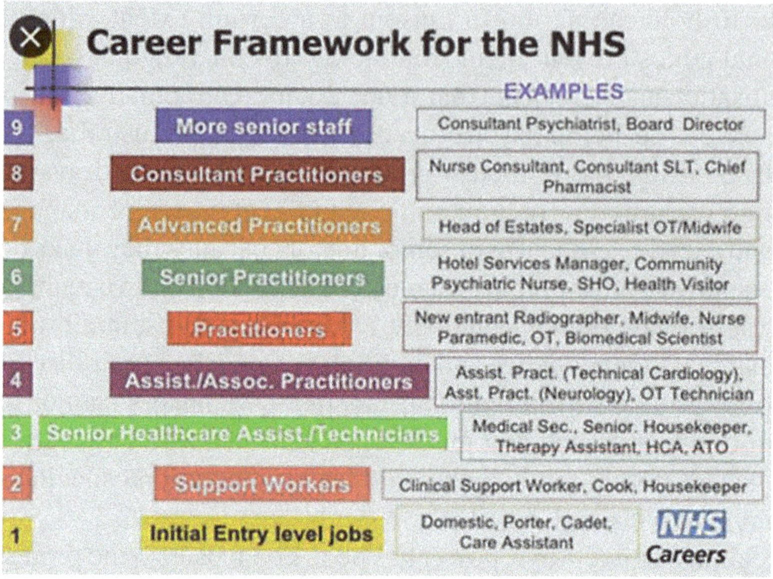

SHORTAGES IN HEALTHCARE WORKERS

Approximately 1.5 million people work in the NHS across the United Kingdom in a wide variety of professions (see Figure 1) (NHS Digital, 2018).

The number of workers has continued to grow, although this growth has not remained in line with demand in either of the four nations of the UK. For example, in England, there was an increase of 18,567 in the number of full-time staff but there were still more than 100,000 vacancies, an increase of 1.8% compared to the previous year. The shortage of nurses is particularly high (41% of all vacancies), followed by administrative and clerical staff (19%) (NHS Digital, 2020). The Royal College of Nursing reported the highest ever vacancy rate in Scotland of 4,000 in 2019 (Royal College of Nursing, 2019a). The extent of the staffing crisis also depends on the region, with Thames Valley reporting the highest shortfall in both medical and non-medical NHS staff (NHS Digital, 2020). According to a recent survey, 40% of consultants in hospitals and 63% of senior doctors reported that they had to manage daily or weekly gaps in senior or junior medical staff (Medical Workforce Unit of the Royal College of Physicians London, 2019). The shortage of frontline staff is particularly significant in the UK compared to other nations. A recent

OECD report noted that the UK has fewer doctors and nurses per head than most other OECD countries. The UK rate is 2.8 doctors and 7.8 nurses per 1,000 population compared to an OECD average of 3.5 and 8.8 respectively (OECD, 2019).

Another cause for concern is staff departures and retention levels. Official NHS figures illustrate the fall in retention levels of NHS staff for British, EU and other non-EU nationals. There have been significant difficulties in retaining UK workers with 136,474 choosing to leave this institution (both on a temporary and permanent basis). The retention rate still remains higher for British citizens (88.4%) compared to EU nationals 83.2% (NHS Digital, 2018)

Table 1. NHS staff departures and retention levels Between June 2016 and June 2017 headcount & percentage

	Leavers	Stability Index
All staff	136,474	88,3%
United Kingdom	109,662	88,4%
European Union	9,854	83,2%
European Economic Area	73	81,1%
Rest of World	8,156	88,7%
Unknown	8,729	90,3%

Source: NHS Digital, NHS Hospital & Community Health Service (HCHS) workforce statistics, 2018

(see Table 1). Such high levels of departure for both categories of workers are a cause for concern because it will no longer be as simple to recruit from other countries in the EU at the end of the transition period following the UK's decision to leave the EU.

According to Rolewicz and Palmer (2019), while many of the shortfalls in staff tend to be filled fairly quickly by temporary staff, there can be a number of problems associated with the dependency on agency staff. Agency staff are more expensive and integrating temporary personnel can disrupt health services and continuity of delivery. Moreover, the inability to fill all the vacancies is having an impact on the quality of care provided. As Buchan, Charlesworth, Gershlick, and Seccombe (2019) argue, the challenge to retain workers is set to increase in the future because the demand for health and social care will continue to increase and thus the need for qualified medical staff. As a House of Commons Health and Social Care Select Committee reported in early 2019 "the nursing workforce is overstretched and struggling to cope with demand" (House of Commons Health Committee, 2018, para.1). Staff shortages are a significant problem across the UK and are putting patients at risk. For example, a shortage of radiologists in Scottish hospitals is currently putting cancer patients at risk. The Scottish Parliament's Cross-Party Group on Cancer reported that 18% of cancer patients in June were not seen within the six-week target because of the shortage (BBC, 2019).

The reason why so many workers are leaving the NHS is because the professional environment has been reported to be deteriorating in recent years. In addition, the chronic shortage of staff means that conditions for those remaining have worsened, thus prompting more staff to leave. In 2018, the public service trade union Unison investigated why NHS workers were leaving, not only drawing on information relayed by their members but also official government data. They explored the reasons for leaving between the financial year 2011/12 and 2017/18. During this period, they noted a 6% increase in the number of staff leaving the NHS. The data showed that one of the major reasons for these departures was to achieve a 'better work-life balance'. Indeed, almost 5,000 staff reported this as a reason for leaving their job. Other reasons cited were lack of opportunities and inadequate pay or benefits. Pay was frozen in the public sector for 2011 and 2012 and then capped to rise only 1% until 2018. Public sector pay has thus not risen in line with inflation overall, meaning a fall in real incomes for public sector workers (HM Treasury, 2018).

Overall, the NHS workforce is more fragmented than ever before. High staff turnover and low morale reported among NHS staff is related to recent pay freezes, under staffing, ever-increasing targets and top-down approaches. The Francis report on the Mid Staffordshire scandal underlined how low staff morale could have a disastrous effect on the provision of good patient care (see Chapter 4 for more details). Personnel are said to be working under increasing pressure. According to an NHS staff survey based on 487,227 staff and 235 NHS trusts in England, the number of staff reporting that they were unwell because of work-related stress stood at 38.4% (Rimmer, 2018).

Even if they do not leave the NHS, the health of the staff is a cause for concern, with a high percentage of days lost as a result of sickness absence. There were more NHS staff taking time off work for illness than ever before in 2017. According to a House of Commons report, health personnel took a total of 16,866,471 sick days off work between 2016 and 2017; a steady rise has been noted since 2012 (Dunne, 2019).

Table 2. Number of days lost in the NHS as a result of sickness absence 2012-2016

Year	Sum of Full-Time Equivalent Sick Days Taken	Sum of Full-Time Equivalent Working Days	Sickness Absence Rate (%)
2012	15,970,492	376,888,359	4.24%
2013	15,424,804	377,092,245	4.09%
2014	16,178,672	384,714,386	4.21%
2015	16,346,443	392,433,945	4.17%
2016	16,866,471	403,377,016	4.18%

Source: NHS Digital 2018

Michelle Sanderson, a paramedic for over 20 years in both the NHS and Royal Air Force (RAF), retired prematurely in 2014 after suffering from Post-Traumatic Stress Disorder (PTSD) and told the press:

There was just far too much to cope with as a paramedic. Working 24-hour shifts, and seeing trauma on a daily basis. You're on standby waiting for that radio to go off – your hyperarousal state and anxiety levels are unbelievable, and that's before you even go on a callout (Kirk 2015, para. 21).

There is also a surprisingly high number of suicides among the nursing profession. According to the Office for National Statistics (ONS), 300 nurses took their own lives between 2011 and 2017 (ONS, 2018a). There are increasing calls for the government to lead a public inquiry into a profession which has a significantly higher rate of suicides than the national average (over 20% higher) (Mitchell, 2019). Nurses are reported to be under increasing pressure because of the rise in demand and staff shortages. According to reports made to the Royal College of Nursing, mental health issues have been repeatedly ignored by employers when staff raised concerns. Nurses are considered to be a key high risk group for suicide due to strain, the responsibility of the profession and the long working hours (Mitchell, 2019).

Kline and Lewis (2018) also point to the disastrous effects of bullying in the NHS. The public sector reports disproportionate bullying and harassment compared to the private sector. Health and social care workers in particular have been subjected to unreasonable management pressure, incivility between co-workers and violent behaviour from patients or relatives of patients. NHS staff surveys showed that 13% of all staff had suffered from bullying or harassment by managers, 18% by co-workers and 28% by patients or relatives of patients (NHS England, 2017). This can have a significant effect on staff turnover. According to some studies, harassment doubles the levels of turnover (Robinson & Perryman, 2004).

Recruiting more staff is thus a priority. The NHS needs to recruit more staff, to improve conditions for health workers and to increase pay. But the future is looking bleak. According to a survey carried out by the General Medical Council in 2018, around a third of the 2,600 doctors interviewed said they were considering reducing hours, a fifth planned to switch to part-time work and a further fifth planned to leave to work abroad. The doctors regretted staff shortages which have made it increasingly difficult to cope with work pressures or ensure the quality of care they would wish to provide (General Medical Council, 2018). Campbell (2018) reports that two in five GPs intend quitting over the next five years. Moreover, the number of GPs taking early retirement has doubled since 2000 (Bostock, 2017). Another problem is the ageing of the nursing profession, a third of whom are aged between 45 and 54 and around 14% over 55. As a significant number of staff take retirement over the next decade, it will add to the problem of recruiting enough staff. NHS England claims that departure of staff could be stemmed if they had better development opportunities and more control over their working lives (NHS England, 2019).

Not only conditions but also how recruitment is managed has also led to an undersupply. The management of the supply of clinical staff is fragmented, involving various departmental bodies, arms-length organisations, healthcare commissioners and providers at both national and local levels, which can lead to uneven supply across the country.

Moreover, it is increasingly costly to train to be a nurse or doctor. In 2017, the government scrapped the bursaries available to nurses to study towards a degree. From August 2017, nursing students started to pay university fees and fees on loans like other students. The rationale behind introducing fees was that it should create more training places because the universities would be able to set their own fees and thus generate more income to create more nursing placements (Health Foundation, 2019). However, it is feared that this measure has discouraged potential nurses from studying and has actually resulted in a decrease in the number of places offered at universities. The number of nursing courses in England fell by 700 places (approximately 23%) between September 2016 and September 2017. However, the government argues the same was true when university fees for other courses were increased in 2012, but places then subsequently increased above the previous threshold. It is thus hoped that the number of places and applicants will recover (Health

Foundation, 2019). Nevertheless, while the government is intent on increasing training places, universities may find it increasingly difficult to provide safe educational supervision for students on placements. Moreover, there seems to be an issue with course acceptance even when students are interested in studying nursing post A-level. A total of 14,000 applicants to nursing were rejected in 2018 (UCAS, 2018). NHS England questions the refusal of thousands of highly motivated and well-qualified applicants at a time when the NHS is significantly understaffed (NHS England, 2019). Furthermore, certain Higher Education Institutions (HEIs) have fixed entry tariffs which are well above the levels set by other HEIs (NHS England, 2019). Doctors also have to pay the exorbitant university fees to train (just over £9,000 per year). The exit of Britain from the EU is likely to further exacerbate the situation.

EU Nationals and Potential Losses Post-Brexit

The tensions surrounding the recruitment of qualified NHS staff have risen since the 2016 referendum results when a majority (51.8%) voted in favour of leaving the EU. Many other sectors, and not just the health sector, are anticipating staffing difficulties because of the high proportion of workers from the EU. Indeed, 14% of workers in the accommodation and food services sector are EU migrants, compared to 5.6% of NHS workers (NHS Digital, 2018). However, in the accommodation and food sector, there is a high turnover within the sector rather than a net loss towards another sector. So while other sectors may be set to lose many workers, they do not have the added problem of British workers also leaving the sector altogether, which is the case in the public health domain.

Support from qualified personnel from other EU countries has been essential for the smooth functioning of the UK public healthcare system. Thanks to the free movement of people within the EU, among the 1.2 million NHS workers, England has 63,650 migrants of European nationality (NHS Digital, 2018). In addition, 80,000 EU nationals work in social care (Department of Health, 2016). Some regions are set to lose more than others, with 11% of EU nationals working for the NHS in London, but only 2% in the North East of England. The percentage is also higher if we consider specific clinical specialties: 10% of hospital doctors and 7% of nurses are reported to be nationals of other EU countries (NHS Digital, 2018). Moreover, 21 trusts report more than a quarter of their staff to be non-British (other EU nationals or non-EU nationals combined) (NHS Digital, 2018).

Figures show an increase in the number of EU nationals coming to work in the NHS between 2009 and 2018. Nationals from the EU-15 (post 2004 countries) increased from 2.2% to 3.8% and those from the Eastern bloc, who entered the EU after 2004, from 0.7% to 1.8% during this period (NHS Digital, 2018). As a House of Commons Library report underlines, the issue with many of the figures relating to departures of EU nationals or increases in the number of EU nationals coming to work in the public health sector in the UK, is that there are a large number of NHS workers for whom the nationality is unaccounted (Baker, 2018). However, in recent years, the number of NHS workers of unknown nationality has been reduced thanks to improved data compilation. Yet this actually raises problems in calculating the increase or decrease of EU nationals working for the NHS and can cause inaccuracies in reporting. In order to improve accuracy, the House of Commons library has thus given figures as a percentage of known categories because the number of workers with unknown nationality was higher in 2016 (just before the referendum) compared to 2018. Nevertheless, it is not possible to be completely accurate on the scale of the change because there are still some staff whose identity remains unknown (and may well be EU migrants too) (Baker, 2018).

Nevertheless, using such a method means that the change in the percentage of EU nationals since the referendum can be calculated with a higher degree of accuracy. According to such calculations and, contrary to a certain number of newspaper articles on this issue, overall there has been very little change in the number of EU staff working for the NHS since June 2016 and, interestingly enough, a slight increase from 5.5% to 5.6%. However, there is a category which has recorded a fall: EU nurses and health visitors. Using the calculation of the percentage of known nationality mentioned above, it is estimated that the number of EU nurses has fallen from 7.4% to 6.8%. This is particularly disconcerting given the shortfall in this category. The percentage of doctors working in the NHS from EU countries other than Britain has remained the same at 9.7% (with a slight initial increase until March 2017) and the percentage of EU clinical support staff has increased from 3.7% to 4.2% (NHS Digital, 2018). Increases and decreases in the number of EU nationals would seem to depend on the country. NHS staff declaring Spanish nationality have fallen from 7,420 to 6,160 (a 15% drop) while the number of Romanians has increased from 3,098 to 4,091 since the 2016 referendum (NHS Digital, 2018). Again these figures need to be treated with a degree of caution because of the fact that there may be Spanish or Romanian staff who have not reported their nationality. For this reason, both absolute numbers

Table 3. Changes in EU staff since June 2016 (headcount basis)

ALL STAFF	Total	EU nationality	Unknown nationality	EU as % of known
Jun 2016	1,164,996	58,698	89,546	**5.5%**
Jun 2018	1,203,610	63,065	71,463	**5.6%**

SCIENTIFIC, THERAPEUTIC AND TECHNICAL	Total	EU nationality	Unknown nationality	EU as % of known
Jun 2016	147,276	6,638	10,605	**4.9%**
Jun 2018	156,345	8,256	8,518	**5.6%**

HOSPITAL DOCTORS	Total	EU nationality	Unknown nationality	EU as % of known
Jun 2016	110,084	10,106	5,812	**9.7%**
Jun 2018	116,191	10,686	5,523	**9.7%**

CLINICAL SUPPORT STAFF	Total	EU nationality	Unknown nationality	EU as % of known
Jun 2016	358,151	11,811	28,348	**3.6%**
Jun 2018	370,192	14,247	22,909	**4.1%**

NURSES AND HEALTH VISITORS	Total	EU nationality	Unknown nationality	EU as % of known
Jun 2016	317,428	21,826	23,536	**7.4%**
Jun 2018	317,884	20,276	17,748	**6.8%**

AMBULANCE STAFF	Total	EU nationality	Unknown nationality	EU as % of known
Jun 2016	19,759	255	3,609	**1.6%**
Jun 2018	21,934	460	3,233	**2.5%**

Source: NHS Digital data, House of Commons Library, Baker, 2018

and percentages of known staff have been given; that is, the percentage out of the total number of staff working for the NHS (see Table 3).

In addition, thousands of EU citizens hold low-level public service positions. These are essential for the proper functioning of health services and for other related services: drivers, housekeepers, cooks, etc. It is worth highlighting the added value to the health sector and more generally to the British economy of EU nationals working in the UK. For example, a study by the University of Oxford showed that EU nationals are more willing to work off-shift schedules (nights, Sundays and public holidays) and adjust more easily to the economy 24/7. That is, an economy that operates 24 hours a day, seven days a week. In addition, they are also on average better educated than natives – almost twice as many are graduates. Indeed, 43% of European nationals have a university degree compared to only 23% of British nationals (Wadsworth, Dhinga, Ottaviano, & Van Reenen, 2016). A study by University College London showed that between 2001 and 2011 the net contribution to public services of EU immigrants was around £22.1 billion, while that of natives was negative, amounting to a deficit of £624.1 billion (Dustmann & Tommaso, 2013). The departure or non-replacement of European nationals or discouraged international workers will most certainly exacerbate the problems in retaining qualified NHS personnel. A shortage of workers in the health sector has the potential to increase costs and the need for expensive temporary employment services.

There is a real cause for concern over a reduced number of EU migrants coming into the UK. The ONS reported that while the number of EU nationals moving to the UK from June 2017 to June 2018 was greater than departures (a net gain of 74,000 EU immigrants), the differences between departures and arrivals was at its lowest level since 2012 (ONS, 2018b). While EU citizens have been guaranteed that they can stay in Britain, there are a number of other reasons, apart from the potential difficulties of remaining legally in the UK post Brexit, which may have resulted in a fall in the net number of EU migrants. The first is the rise in xenophobia, unleashed by the debate on Brexit, which is likely to have dissuaded skilled workers from coming to work in a country where the climate has become more hostile to foreign workers, which is also true for all foreign workers. As the Labour Exploitation Advisory Group explained:

A rise in hate crime and hostility post referendum contributes to a general sense of being unwelcome and makes migrant workers feel like 'second class citizens' in the UK. This undermines confidence in rights and makes it more difficult to speak out about poor treatment (Labour Exploitation Advisory Group, 2017, p. 1).

The relative growth of other EU economies could also be the reason why there is a fall in the net number of EU migrants coming to Britain. Indeed, Spain is a case in point. After the 2009 financial crisis and the severe recession that ensued, Spanish nationals started to migrate to find work elsewhere in Europe, but with improved conditions they can now find work more easily in their country of origin. It is therefore very difficult to directly relate the fall in the number of EU workers in the NHS to the Brexit effect. The decline in the number of EU migrants working for the NHS could also be for the same reasons as for British nationals described above; that is, increased stress and deteriorating working standards.

Yet the full effect of Brexit on the retention rate of EU migrants in the NHS is still to be seen because the UK is still in the transition period. If there is no longer freedom of movement of people from other EU countries, then the number of EU migrants coming to work in the UK in the future is certainly likely to decline. As Britain becomes an even more hostile place to work and immigration policies post-Brexit deter EU nationals from coming to the UK, there will most certainly be a reduction in the number of EU nationals.

Notwithstanding the reliance on EU nationals, the NHS actually relies more on nationals from outside the EU. Foreign nationals account for 12.5% of NHS employees (139,000 workers). While as a region, the EU is the most highly represented (62,000) or 5.6%, 45,000 employees come from Asia and 21,000 from Africa. The most highly represented single nationality is Indian

(19,142), then Philipine (16,807) ahead of Irish (13,132), Polish (8,896), Portuguese (6,899) and Spanish (6,160) (NHS Digital, 2018).

However, there is particular concern that stringent immigration laws will make it very difficult to continue to recruit EU workers once they are subject to the same conditions as other immigrants. Until June 2018, the strict immigration quotas meant that doctors wishing to come to the UK from non-EU countries were restricted in number because of a cap on visas given to skilled workers (so called tier 2 visas). The UK is even more reliant on foreign doctors than any other category of worker. However, owing to the cap on skilled workers, 1,518 applications for visas by foreign doctors were turned down in the first quarter of 2018. There has been a fall from 30% to 26% of non-British doctors which could be in part related to these more stringent immigration conditions (BMA, 2019).

SOLVING THE STAFFING CRISIS

In recent years, a number of measures have been put in place to try and solve the staffing crisis. The government pledged extra money to fill the gap in funding in the NHS in the 2017 and 2018 Autumn Statements, with extra funding to rise to £20.5 billion in 2023/24. However, this money was directed at front-line NHS services and excluded some other vital areas in desperate need of funding such as workforce training (Health Foundation, 2019). The government did promise a 25% rise in NHS training placements and university placements in 2017 and 2018 following the recommendations of NHS England. From 2020/21, NHS England also announced it would provide funding for clinical placements for as many places as universities could fill, up to a 50% increase. Every nurse or midwife graduating has also been offered a five-year NHS job guarantee provided they take up the position in the region in which they qualify (NHS England, 2019). NHS England has promised to make training more accessible with a special new NHS online nursing degree with placements within NHS trusts and primary care units, which is expected to be available towards the end of 2020.

In the lead up to the 2019 general elections, the Conservative Party promised a pay rise of at least 6.5% for one million NHS employees - nurses, midwives and cleaners. It also announced the creation of 50,000 additional nursing posts and a student grant to encourage further study in this field (Conservative Party, 2019). The Conservative Party has committed to reintroducing the NHS scholarship scheme to help train and recruit 50,000 nurses. It also pledged to open five new medical schools to train the next generation of NHS staff, and to hire an extra 6,000 GPs, to create 550 million general surgery appointments and 50 million GP appointments per year, an increase of more than 15% (Conservative Party, 2019). While the proposal to increase the number of doctors and nurses is commendable, it should be noted that the training of doctors and nurses will take years and no budget has been clearly presented to fund this increase in staff and the training of health professionals. Paradoxically, it was the Conservative Chancellor of the Exchequer, George Osborne, who put an end to the payment of scholarships and tuition fees for nurses in 2015. The Royal College of Nursing says that attempts to compensate for the shortage of staff are not enough. It argues that more ambitious plans are needed to address NHS staff shortages. Moreover, the Conservative manifesto for 2019 does not propose to remove all nursing fees. The Conservative government will maintain tuition fees, which are very high (Royal College of Nursing, 2019b). Dave Prentis, General Secretary of Unison, said:

No one should be fooled by the promises for the NHS and public sector. For the past nine years the Tories have slashed funding and let services slide. Now they are trumpeting a reversal of their own bungled policy of scrapping the nursing bursary – a problem of their own making (Unison, 2019, para. 3-4)

In Scotland and Wales where the bursaries have been maintained for nurses, there was an increase in the number of trainees by 9.3% in Scotland and 6.2% in Wales (Buchan et al., 2019).

Another response to the shortage of staff owing to significant university fees has been the introduction of new routes for nursing, such as nursing associates, nursing degree apprenticeships and Nurse First Schemes. In January 2019, the first nursing associates joined the nursing team to provide care and treatment in a wide range of health and care settings. The intention was to address a skills gap between unregulated health and care assistants and registered nurses (Mitchell, 2019). The government is encouraging the creation of apprenticeships and nursing schemes for both nursing associates and standard nursing training in order to remove the burden of paying fees from the trainee. However, according to the Chief Executive of Health Education in England, this has actually had unintended consequences; it has triggered a transfer of social care staff into nursing training (Longhurst, 2018).

On account of the difficulty in recruiting non-British staff once Britain leaves the EU, there has been increasing pressure on the government to make it easier to recruit NHS staff from overseas. In June 2018, the home secretary Sajid Javid confirmed that the government would relax the cap on skilled workers, specifically for medical professionals (Home Office, 2018). The then Health and Social Care secretary Jeremy Hunt recognised the importance of this measure and the contribution of overseas staff:

Overseas staff have been a vital part of our NHS since its creation 70 years ago. Today's news sends a clear message to nurses and doctors from around the world that the NHS welcomes and values their skills and dedication. It's fantastic that patients will now benefit from the care of thousands more talented staff (Home Office, 2018, para. 10).

Moreover, to address the shortage of staff, the 2019 Conservative manifesto also proposed the introduction of an immigration system which would allow doctors and nurses from around the world to come to work in the UK after Brexit, using NHS visas and a points-based immigration system (Conservative Party, 2019). More specifically, the UK policy statement in January 2020 underlined how this system would work at the end of the transition period. It states that free movement will end and an Immigration Bill will be introduced after the transition period on the basis of a fair points-based system. The aim of this bill is to attract high-skilled workers for the economy, community and to work in public services. It is based on skills and not place of origin. It states that from 1 January 2021, EU and non-EU citizens will be treated equally with priority to the highest skills and the greatest talents: scientists, engineers, academics and other highly-skilled workers. However, there will also be a low-skilled or temporary work route, which could fill vacancies and help relieve pressure in key sectors (which will be monitored regularly). Salary thresholds have been set at £30,000 and £25,600 (Home Office, 2020). However, such thresholds were criticised because a number of vital NHS workers (international workers) earn less, so this may suggest why the policy statement includes the following:

Under the points-based system for skilled workers, applicants will be able to 'trade' characteristics such as their specific job offer and qualifications against a lower salary (...) there will continue to be different arrangements for a small number of occupations where the salary threshold will be based on published pay scales. We will set the requirements for new entrants 30% lower than the rate for experienced workers in any occupation and only use the base salary (and not the allowances or pension contributions) to determine whether the salary threshold is met (Home Office, 2020, para.4).

In addition, applicants have to demonstrate they have a job offer from an approved sponsor and that this job fills the aforementioned requirements.

While some similar measures might have been taken in any case given staff shortages in the NHS, future considerations on being able to continue to recruit new staff from EU countries weighed even more heavily on this decision. However, the future obligation for EU citizens to have to apply for a visa to work may be dissuasive despite such measures. It has also been important to reassure EU migrants currently working in the UK that they can stay. The UK Government has sent clear messages that the legal rights of EU nationals living in the UK will be properly protected. Amidst great uncertainty which perhaps encouraged some to leave the UK before this notice was issued, the Home Office sent a letter to EU citizens to reassure them that their right to remain in the UK would be safeguarded (HM Government, 2018). This move was very important because there was a degree of uncertainty about whether European citizens currently resident in the UK could benefit from the Vienna Convention on the Law of Treaties of 1989, which stipulates that the acquired rights of individuals cannot be withdrawn if new treaties between countries are signed.

Beyond measures to retain EU workers, there is also a move to try to reduce the dependency on foreign workers and recruit more British workers. A House of Lords Select Committee on the Long-Term Sustainability of the NHS report notes that there has been a long-standing reliance on foreign nationals in the NHS (House of Lords, 2017). The committee states that the long-term solution is for the government to ensure the supply of well-trained health and social care workers from within the country. The report noted an absence of a national long-term strategy which could secure the necessary trained staff needed in health and social care over the next 10 to15 years. They pointed to the fragmented nature of staff planning across the country as an issue still to be solved (House of Lords, 2017).

In light of such retention problems and, on the request of the Secretary of State for Health, the NHS Improvement set up a national retention programme specifically targeting NHS trusts where there was a low rate of retention. It rolled out the programme in 2017, in association with NHS employers (NHS Improvement, 2019). The programme was designed to support hospital trusts to make the NHS a better place to work. Support included schemes for NHS workers beginning their career, better use of expertise of experienced workers, more flexibility for work shifts and support for career development (NHS Improvement, 2019). The initial targets were those trusts with the highest turnover rates. Gradually, the scheme was rolled out in other hospitals (in total 140). Focus groups of HR nursing leaders also shared their experiences and best practices in retention. NHS Improvement has reported that progress has been made since the programme began in June 2017. In England, national nursing staff turnover rates have been reduced from 12.5% to 11.9% (NHS Improvement, 2019).

Finally, in order to identify present and future staff challenges, NHS staff are invited to take part in an annual survey. The survey is centred around four main criteria: appraisal and development, health and wellbeing, staff engagement and involvement and raising concerns. The most recent staff survey identified a number of areas where progress had been made and highlighted ongoing challenges. The survey found that there has been positive progress in people management including in line management skills. However, health and wellbeing, staff engagement and scores for bullying and harassment have not improved. Nevertheless, the percentage of staff who recommended the organisation as a place to work rose slightly from the previous year to 63% (up 1.7% from 2018). More staff felt valued by their organisation, although there was still not a majority of staff who reported feeling valued (48%). On a positive note, 74% felt enthusiastic about their jobs. In terms of retention levels, the overall percentage of staff reporting that they were considering leaving the organisation fell slightly on previous years but was still high (21%) (NHS Employers 2020).

CONCLUSION

Frontline professionals but also ancillary staff are essential to the running of the NHS. A number of governance challenges have been underlined in this chapter. While training staff is important, creating commitment, whether it be from staff born in the UK or from overseas, is also essential. Increased uncertainty and the added pressures of the profession is making this very difficult. The lack of effective policies to support training of UK professionals until very recently and the declining attractiveness of the profession mean that more needs to be done to train and retain NHS workers, especially faced with the potential loss of overseas staff post-Brexit. While most NHS institutions across the UK have a staff governance framework in place to ensure staff are treated well, research has shown that the deteriorating conditions mean that more effective governance frameworks to manage staff are needed in the NHS. In addition to the above pressures, NHS clinicians are also increasingly accountable to the service user, which we will consider next.

REFERENCES

Alford, R. (1975). *Healthcare politics*. University of Chicago Press.

Baker, C. (2018, October 10). *NHS staff from oversea: Statistics*. Briefing Paper. No 773810. House of Commons Library. Retrieved February 3, 2019, from https://commonslibrary.parliament.uk/ research-briefings/cbp-7783/

BBC News. (2016, April 6). *Junior doctors' row: The dispute explained*. Retrieved February 28, 2019, from https://www.bbc.co.uk/news/health-34775980

BBC News. (2019, November 9). *NHS staff shortages put cancer survival rates at risk*. Retrieved February 28, 2019, from https://www.bbc.com/news/uk-scotland-50454018

BMA. (2013). *Red tape and lack of capacity prevent doctors from making NHS improvements*. Retrieved January 6, 2014, from https://www.bma.org.uk/nhsworking

BMA. (2019, May 16). *Visa cap blocks thousands of medical applications*. Retrieved January 22, 2019, https://www.bma.org.uk/ news/2018/may/ visa-cap-blocks-thousands-of- medical-applications

Bostock, N. (2017, April 5). GP early retirements have doubled since start of the decade. *GP*. Retrieved January 3, 2019, from www.gponline.com/gp-early-retirements-doubled-start-decade/article/1461188

Buchan, J., Charlesworth, A., Gershlick, B., & Seccombe, I. (2019). *A critical moment: NHS staffing trends and retention and attrition*. The Health Foundation. Retrieved January 7, 2020, from https://reader.health.org.uk/a-critical-moment/executive-summary-trends-in-the-nhs-workforce

Campbell, D. (2018, May 31). Two in five GPs in England intend to quit within five years – survey. *The Guardian*. Retrieved January 7, 2019, from www.theguardian.com/ society/2018/may/31/ two-in-five-gps-in-england-intend-to-quit-within-five-years-survey

Conservative Party. (2019). *The Conservative and Unionist Party Manifesto 2019*. Retrieved January 3, 2020, from https://general-election-2010.co.uk/ 2019-general-election-manifestos/ conservative-manifesto-2019.pdf

Cox, D. (2001). Dilemmas in healthcare management. In C. Komaromy (Ed.), *Dilemmas in UK healthcare* (pp. 41–62). Open University Press.

Dayan, M., & Edwards, N. (2017). *Learning from Scotland's NHS*. Nuffield Trust. Retrieved February 5, 2020, from https://www.nuffieldtrust.org.uk/ research/learning-from-scotland-s-nhs

Dunne, P. (2017, June 21). *NHS Lost working days. Written question – 335*. Retrieved January, 18, 2019, from https://www.parliament.uk/ business/ publications/ written-questions-answers-statements/ written-question/ Commons/2017-06-21/335/

Dustmann, C., & Fratini, T. (2014, November). The fiscal effects of immigration to the UK. *Economic Journal (London), 124*(580), F593–F643. doi:10.1111/ ecoj.12181

General Medical Council. (2018). *The state of medical education and practice in the UK*. General Medical Council.

HM Government. (2018, December). *The UK's future skills-based immigration system*. CM972. Crown.

Ham, C. (2009). *Health policy in Britain* (6th ed.). Palgrave Macmillan. doi:10.1007/978-1-137-01397-2

Health Foundation. (2018, June 16). *Health Foundation response to government announcement of additional NHS funding*. The Health Foundation. Retrieved January 22, 2019, from https://www.health.org.uk/ news-and-comment/news/ health-foundation-response-to- government-announcement-of- additional-nhs-funding

HM Treasury. (2018 July 24). Around one million public sector workers to get pay rise. *HM Treasury*. Retrieved January 21, 2019, from https://www.gov.uk/ government/news/ around-one-million-public-sector-workers-to-get-pay-rise

Home Office. (2018, June 15). Doctors and nurses to be taken out of Tier 2 visa *cap. Home Office*. Retrieved January 22, 2019, from https://www.gov. uk/ government/news/ doctors-and-nurses-to-be-taken-out-of-tier-2-visa-cap

Home Office. (2020, February 19). Policy Paper: The UK's points-based immigration system: policy statement. *Home Office*. Retrieved March 24, 2020, from https://www.gov.uk/government/ publications/the-uks-points-based-immigration-system-policy-statement/ the-uks-points-based-immigration-system-policy-statement

House of Commons Health Committee. (2018). *The nursing workforce: Second report of session 2017–19*. TSO. The Stationery Office.

House of Lords. (2017, April 5). *The long-term sustainability of the NHS and adult social care*. Committee Office.

Kirk, A. (2015, April 25). Paramedics take 40,000 days off sick with stress as strain on NHS takes toll. *The Guardian*. Retrieved April 7, 2017, from https://www.theguardian.com/ society/2015/apr/25/ paramedics-take-40000-days-off-sick-with-stress-nhs-demand

Klein, R. (2013). *The new politics of the NHS: From creation to reinvention* (3rd ed.). Radcliffe Publishing.

Kline, R., & Lewis, D. (2018, October 24). The price of fear: Estimating the financial cost of bullying and harassment to the NHS in England. *Public Money and Management*. Retrieved January 21, 2019, from https://www.tandfonline.com/doi/full/10.1080/09540962.2018.1535044

Labour Exploitation Advisory Group. (2017, August) *Lost in transition, Brexit and labour exploitation*. FLEX & the Labour Exploitation Advisory Group. Retrieved January 21, 2019, from https://www.labourexploitation.org/ publications/lost-transition-brexit-labour-exploitation

Longhurst, C. (2018, June 19). Nursing associate role 'has made things worse for social care'. *Nursing Standard*. Retrieved April 4, 2020, from https://rcni.com/ nursing-standard/newsroom/news/ nursing-associate-role-has-made-things-worse-social-care-135056

Medical Workforce Unit of the Royal College of Physicians London. (2019, October 3). Focus on physicians: 2018-2019 census (UK consultants and higher specialty trainees). *Royal College of Physicians*. Retrieved April 4, 2020, from https://www.rcplondon.ac.uk/ projects/outputs/ focus-physicians-2018-19-census-uk- consultants-and-higher-specialty-trainees

Mitchell, G. (2019, 29 April). Figures spark call for inquiry into 'alarming' levels of nurse suicide. *Nursing Times*. Retrieved April 4, 2020, from https://www.nursingtimes.net/ news/workforce/figures- spark-call-for-inquiry-into-alarming-levels-of-nurse-suicide-29-04-2019/

NHS Digital. (2018). *NHS Hospital & Community Health Service (HCHS) workforce statistics*. Retrieved March 6, 2019, from https://digital.nhs.uk/ data-and-information/publications/ statistical/nhs-workforce-statistics

NHS Digital. (2020, February 27). *NHS vacancy statistics England February 2015 - December 2019, experimental statistics*. Retrieved April 5, 2020, from https://digital.nhs.uk/ data-and-information/publications/ statistical/nhs-vacancies-survey/ february-2015---december-2019-experimental-statistics

NHS Employers. (2020, February 19). *NHS staff survey 2019 - progress and challenges*. Retrieved April 6, 2020, from https://www.nhsemployers.org/ retention-and-staff-experience/ staff-engagement/the-nhs-staff-survey/ nhs-staff-survey-2019

NHS England. (2017). *NHS staff surveys*. Retrieved April 3, 2020, from www.nhsstaffsurveys.com/Page/1064/Latest- Results/2017-Results

NHS England. (2019). *The NHS long-term plan*. London: NHS England. Retrieved February 3, 2020, from https://www.longtermplan.nhs.uk/ publication/nhs-long-term-plan/

NHS Improvement. (2019). *The national retention programme: Two years on*. Retrieved February 3, 2020, from https://improvement.nhs.uk/resources/ national-retention-programme-two-years-on/

OECD. (2019). *Health at a glance*. OECD.

ONS. (2018a, October 24). *Suicide deaths among nurses aged 20 to 64 years, deaths registered in England and Wales between 2011 and 2017*. ONS. Retrieved April 3, 2020, from https://www.ons.gov.uk/ peoplepopulationandcommunity/ birthsdeathsandmarriages/ deaths/ adhocs/009209 suicidedeathsamongnursesaged 20to64yearsdeathsregisteredin englandandwalesbetween2011and2017

ONS. (2018b, November). *Migration Statistics Quarterly Report*. ONS. Retrieved January 21, 2019, from https://www.ons.gov.uk/ peoplepopulationandcommunity/ populationandmigration/ internationalmigration/ bulletins/migrationstatistics quarterlyreport/ november2018

Rimmer, A. (2018, March 6). Staff stress levels reflect rising pressures on NHS, says NHS leaders. *BMJ*, *360*. Retrieved January 4, 2019, from https://www.ncbi.nlm.nih.gov/pubmed/29511003

Robinson, D., & Perryman, S. (Eds.). (2004). *Healthy attitudes: Quality of working life in the London NHS 2000–2002*. Institute of Employment Studies.

Rolewicz, L., & Palmer, B. (2019). *The NHS workforce in numbers*. Nuffield Trust. Retrieved on April 4, 2020, from https://www.nuffieldtrust.org.uk/resource/the-nhs-workforce-in-numbers

Royal College of Nursing. (2019a, September 3). NHS Scotland nursing vacancies reach all time high. *Royal College of Nursing*. Retrieved January 24, 2020 from https://www.rcn.org.uk/news-and-events/news/isd-workforce-stats-3-sept-2019

Royal College of Nursing. (2019b, November 24). Royal College of Nursing responds to Conservative Party general election manifesto. *Royal College of Nursing*. Retrieved January 24, 2020, from https://www.rcn.org.uk/news-and-events/press-releases/Conservative

Unison. (2019, November 24). Tories are offering nothing new. *Unison*. Retrieved April 5, 2020, from https://www.unison.org.uk/news/2019/11/tories-offering-nothing-new/

Universities and Colleges Admissions Service (UCAS). (2018). *Daily Clearing Analysis: Overview. Nursing analysis at 00:05 on Thursday 13 September 2018 (28 days after A level results day).* Retrieved September 6, 2018, from https://www.ucas.com/file/187976/download?token=7mXkvYI3

Wadsworth, J., Dhinga, S., Ottaviano, G., & Van Reenen, J. (2016). *Brexit and the impact of immigration on the UK. CEP Brexit Analysis n° 5*. London School of Economics.

ENDNOTE

1 The Scottish governance framework is considered in more detail in Chapter 5.

Chapter 4
Personal and Public Involvement in Healthcare Provision

ABSTRACT

Personal and public involvement in healthcare provision has become an essential part of the governance framework of the National Health Service (NHS) today. Patient safety, quality, and responsiveness of care are the main priorities of national healthcare providers. Yet in practice, there are significant limitations to the introduction of a true patient- or person-centred approach, which will be described in this chapter. Two case studies have been included to illustrate the challenges to implementing a true person-centred approach in the NHS. The first relates to the Mid-Staffordshire Hospital Trust where hundreds of patients died as a result of sub-standard levels of care. The second focuses on a family's struggle to access a joined-up package of care for a Parkinson's disease sufferer in a primary care setting.

INTRODUCTION

In recent years, the involvement of the patient in the process of treating and providing greater choice to the individual has become an important part of healthcare practice in the UK. The governance of the National Health Service (NHS) is increasingly about co-production and granting the patient and public (family or advocate) an active role in healthcare provision. The

DOI: 10.4018/978-1-7998-3928-6.ch004

clinical governance framework introduced by New Labour in the late 1990s ensured that the patient-centred or person-centred approach was at the very heart of public healthcare provision. Although there is no widely accepted definition, person-centred care can be defined as a holistic approach to meet the needs and priorities of the person receiving healthcare ahead of all other stakeholders of the system (health professionals, etc.). Starfield (2011) underlines the subtle difference between patient and person-centred care. While patient-centred care tends to focus on care of diseases (generally chronic), person-focused or centred care is provided to patients over time, independent of care for particular diseases. However, in practice NHS documents tend to mix the two. Mead and Bower (2000), after an extensive literature review, underline five key components that make up patient-centred care: patient-as-person (focusing on the patient as a person); sharing power and responsibility (creating an egalitarian relationship between patient and providers, informing the patient and family and allowing the patient to choose…); therapeutic alliance (emphasis on empathy and respect; and doctor-as-person (clinical encounter). Personal and Public Involvement (PPI) is also at the heart of the health governance framework. PPI can be described as the active and effective involvement of service users, carers and the public in Health and Social Care (HSC) services. Yet in practice, there are significant limitations to the introduction of a true PPI, patient- or person-centred approach, which will be described in this chapter. Two case studies also included here illustrate the challenges of implementing a true person-centred approach in the NHS.

THE ORIGINS OF PATIENT- OR PERSON-CENTRED HEALTHCARE

The Health Foundation has traced the origins of person-centred healthcare and attributed this expression to psychologist Carl Rogers (1951) who used the term in relation to psychotherapy. In the late 1970s, the American psychiatrist George Engel promoted a bio-psychosocial model of health; that is a person-centred model of healthcare. It is not necessarily the definition adopted by the NHS today but it did put focus on the need for empathy and for the professional to be prepared to suspend judgment and appreciate the services user's or patient's perspective (The Health Foundation, 2013).

The World Health Organisation (WHO) explains that while there have been significant health improvements over the last century, despite increasing health expenditure and advances in health services, people are not really any healthier in body or mind and they are not on the whole any happier with the health services they receive. However, patient safety and quality and responsiveness of care should be a national health provider's priority. In order to ensure a people-centred approach to healthcare within the governance framework of health services, the WHO has called upon governments to take into consideration the rights and needs as well as the responsibilities and capacities of all health constituents and stakeholders (WHO, 2007). The organisation thus prepared a framework for 'people-centred health' to ensure the inclusion of the patients themselves. The statement was endorsed by WHO Member States during the 58th session of the Regional Committee for the Western Pacific, held in the Republic of Korea in September 2007. Such a framework sets some general principles and guidance for countries to take policy reforms at the national and local level in order to ensure the provision of people-centred health services.

Healthcare providers are increasingly called upon to take into account the demands of the patient through a person-centred approach. In the UK, action to be more inclusive of patients preceded the WHO prescription for person-centred health with the introduction of the Patient Charter in 1991 in England. The Charter set specific rights for patients and key targets that providers must achieve. Indeed, rights included that of receiving emergency medical care at any time through a General Practitioner (GP) or through emergency ambulance services and a hospital accident and emergency (A&E) department; the right to be referred to a consultant who is acceptable to a patient, when a GP thinks this is necessary, and to be able to get a second opinion if a patient and GP agree this to be desirable; the right to a clear explanation of any treatment proposed and the right to be given detailed information on local health services, including quality standards and maximum waiting times. The 1995 updated and enlarged Patient's Charter set forth new standards and targets to be achieved, including 90% of outpatients to be seen within 13 weeks for the first appointment and 100% within 26 weeks, a three to four-hour standard for 'trolley waits' in A&E departments, reduced to two hours in April 1996 (Ham, 2009). UK health policy prescriptions have thus incorporated the notion of person-centredness. The Patient's Charter was then supplemented by the NHS Plan 2000 and subsequently replaced by the NHS Constitution for England in 2013.

The introduction of clinical governance in the late 1990s as described in Chapter 1 was also instrumental for patient inclusiveness. Under clinical governance guidelines, NHS service providers are accountable for improving the quality of their services and safeguarding high standards of care. One of the key components of this new approach is patient involvement. The introduction of clinical governance which enhances patient involvement was in response to a number of failures in standards of NHS care and, more generally, criticism of the professionally dominated and insular approach of health professionals towards patients. The commitment to a patient-centred approach under Tony Blair's government has led to a number of further commitments. For example, the creation of the Quality and Outcomes Framework, whose underlying aim is to ensure that individuals monitor and maintain their own health. The clinical governance framework imposes a duty on NHS organisations and their staff to continually improve the quality of patient care.

Under the Health and Social Care Act of 2012, NHS England and Clinical Commissioning Groups (CCGs) have a legal duty to involve patients in their care (The Health Foundation, 2013). The Care Act of 2014 also calls on local authorities and health organisations to ensure that individuals receiving care are actively encouraged and supported to participate and are able to design care and support based around achievement of their goals.

PATIENT INCLUSIVENESS WITHIN THE NHS IN PRACTICE

A number of policies have been rolled out to include patients in the delivery of healthcare. Clinical governance has thus evolved to encompass using patient and public inclusive policies to deal with poor practitioner performance and to try to learn from adverse events and errors (Department of Health, 1999; Department of Health, 2000).

Part of the clinical governance framework as shown in the diagram in Figure 1 is patient and public involvement (PPI). PPI is more commonly used to involve the patient in research processes. However, within the clinical governance framework, it refers to everyone who uses services, which includes not only the patient but also carers and families. Participation or engagement and involvement, according to NHS England, may be varied whether it be through social media, voluntary community and social enterprise organisation, elected representatives, formal consultations and meetings. The NHS thus pledges to work in partnership with patients and the public to improve patient safety, patient experience and health outcomes (NHS England, 2017). NHS England provides a list of ways in which the patient and public are included in public health service delivery: public board meetings, committees,

Figure 1. Clinical governance framework in the NHS
Source: Department of Health (2001)

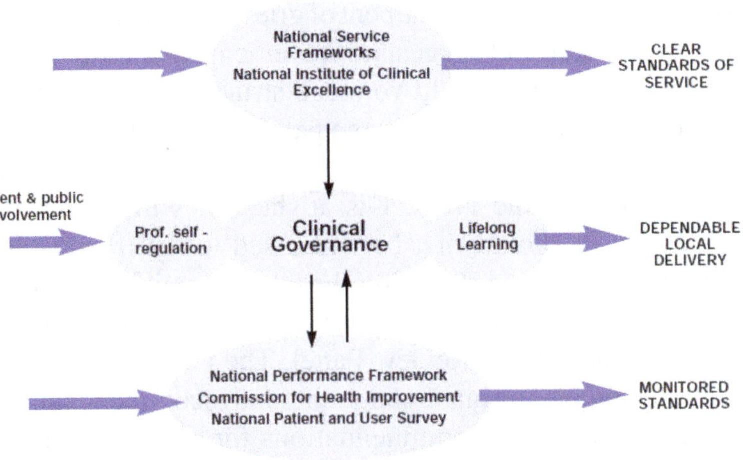

representatives of patients and the public, called PPV partners, NHS citizens' dialogue groups, etc.

Moreover, a number of different methods are currently in place within the NHS which actively encourage patients to judge the provision of health by sharing their experiences of care and treatment, completing surveys, etc. Testimonials are also a way of evaluating the provision of healthcare and are posted regularly on NHS websites (Patient Opinion, NHS Choices, etc.), and also on special care and charity websites. Stories told by individuals from their own perspective and in a healthcare setting can provide healthcare providers with an opportunity to understand experiences of care and to gain an insight into what could be done to improve the patient's experience. Providing an outlet for patients to complain can be a useful way of not only ensuring that individual rights to quality healthcare are respected but also of increasing awareness of safety-related problems within health organisations, or various problems relating to healthcare delivery.

All NHS healthcare organisations in England and Scotland must carry out postal surveys to give patients a chance to air their views on their recent experience of healthcare. These national surveys aim to compare results locally and should enable policy makers and regulators to improve services. In addition, the complaints system has also gradually been improved, especially from 1996 onwards. Since 1985, the Hospital Complaints Procedure Act set forth a number of national procedures for hospitals to deal with complaints.

Complaints regarding GPs are made to the Family Health Services Authority (FHSA). From the 1990s, complaints procedures were improved because of criticism of the lack of effective treatment of grievances. The Wilson committee was set up to investigate and suggest improvements to the complaints system and, in 1994, a more simplified two-stage structure system for grievances was introduced. In 1996, in line with the patient-centred approach, a unified complaints system was introduced for hospitals, community health services and family services in the NHS. Dissatisfaction with acute, primary or secondary healthcare should first be addressed to the trust, CCG or other care provider with a view to resolving the issue as quickly as possible (by a Local Resolutions Unit). However, if the complaint is unresolved, it is then addressed to an Independent Review Panel. The panel must investigate the complaint, write a report and make comments and recommendations to redress the grievance and/or make recommendations for service improvements. If this review is not satisfactory, then the complainant can refer the matter to the Health Service Commissioner at NHS England (Department of Health, 2010). The latter then publishes an annual overview and six-monthly reports on investigations into complaints with possible recommendations for action. Beyond providing a system for complaints, the NHS also actively encourages patients to give their views on the health system.

The NHS Patient Experience Framework underlines that patient experience is one of the central outcomes to be considered along with effectiveness and safety (The Health Foundation, 2013). The NHS Future Forum called for the establishment of new metrics to bring together already existing data on patient experience. The NHS has taken several initiatives to enable the patient to share his or her experience of healthcare provision and in so doing evaluate the quality of care provided. The NHS Constitution and the Health Act of January 2010 impose a legal obligation on service providers to take into account the decisions and actions of patient experience. The NHS Outcomes Framework also makes clear that the provision of a good experience of care for patients is a fundamental part of the NHS. The NHS Patient Experience Framework sets forth a definition and measurement of patients' experiences. Patient-Reported Experience Measures (PREMs) and Patient-Reported Outcomes (PROMS) are also currently used by NHS providers. The Department of Health has been active in promoting a patient- or person-centred approach. The 2010 White Paper, *Equity and Excellence: Liberating the NHS* (Department of Health, 2010) underlines that there should be more emphasis on improving people's experience of healthcare. In 2013, a Department of Health Review Team set up a dedicated postal and email address for people to send accounts and experiences of healthcare. They received 2,500 letters and emails and the team reviewed the data. Seven public engagement events were also held. The review team visited nine NHS hospitals and one hospice to meet up with complaints managers, frontline staff and board members (Department of Health, 2013).

Some hospital trusts and GP practices routinely seek out more general feedback: how long a patient has been waiting, quality of care, etc. Many trusts also have a specialised complaints department. Moreover, national bodies support quality improvement through patient input such as Healthwatch England, Citizens Advice, Patients Association, Actions for Victims of Medical Accidents, the Consumers Association, National Voices, etc. (The Health Foundation, 2013). In England, an annual General Practice Patient Survey is carried out to collate information on people's experience of primary care. It surveys five million people each year. For hospitals, a National Adult Inpatient Survey has been in place since 2002 which surveys 600,000 patients every year (The Health Foundation, 2013).

The UK also has a number of websites where patients and family members can post their stories about NHS care experiences. For example, Patient Opinion invites patients and families to post short anonymous stories and 45,000 testimonials are available on the website. Once the stories are published, the website administrators contact the relevant health organisation giving them an opportunity to post a reply. The Francis Report (Francis, 2013) claims that this site has the potential to improve the quality of care. NHS Choices is another website which provides patients with the opportunity to give accounts of service provision, particularly in a hospital setting. Comments often relate to human errors, incorrect medical recording and medical errors, etc. (The Health Foundation, 2013).

The Legal Framework for Patient Protection

Since there has been an increase in the reporting of adverse effects, that is people dying or being seriously injured, it would seem important to take criticisms of health services made by patients and the general public seriously. Indeed 400 people have been reported as dying or being seriously injured after the use of medical devices in the NHS, 10,000 people had adverse reactions to drugs prescribed by NHS consultants and 1,150 people committed suicide despite being in contact with NHS mental health services. The NHS receives roughly 28,000 written complaints a year on clinical treatment in hospital and pays £400 million in clinical negligence claims (Reader, Gillespie, & Roberts, 2013). Adverse effects have been reported to be higher in Great Britain (around 10%) than France, for example (3.7%) (Guiliani, Gault, Fares, Jegu, Eleni, Biga, & Vidal-Trecan, 2009). A series of investigations and reports which examine patient complaints and testimonials on care emphasise the importance of using such material to drive improvements in healthcare: The Wilson Report *Being Heard* of May 1994, the Public Law Project's report *Cause for Complaint*? of September 1999 and the York Health Economics Consortium's report (*The York Report*) published in March 2001 are just some examples of work in this area. These reports have been instrumental in improving the complaints procedure and the development of a person-centred or patient-centred approach within the NHS.

The NHS is thus heavily scrutinised by civil society and a number of legal challenges against the NHS or NHS practitioners make the front pages of newspapers. An overriding issue that tends to affect most front-line staff is the fear of finding themselves in breach of their various legal duties. In the event of death of a patient, a GP or a hospital trust may be accused of sub-standard care. For example, in 2015, Dr Hadiza Bawa-Garba was found guilty of manslaughter by gross negligence at the Criminal Court of Justice after the death of a six-year-old Down's syndrome patient who died 11 hours after being admitted to hospital following a heart attack. More generally, the NHS pays a significant amount in personal injuries. In 2017/8, the NHS paid out over £1.63 billion in damages to claimants, which represents an increase of 33% on the previous year (NHS Resolution, 2018).

Lawson (2015) explains that CCGs are also facing more and more legal challenges as budgets have been squeezed and information technology has forced decision making to become more transparent. As mentioned previously, rationing is increasingly more evident in decision processes in deciding whether treatment should be funded or not. However, CCGs do have a duty under the National Health Service Act 2006 to meet 'reasonable requirements' for healthcare. Although it is the CCGs role to consider what is reasonable, their decision can be overturned in law courts, especially if the treatment has been recommended by NICE and the CCG refuses to supply it. For example, in 2014, a CCG refused to fund egg freezing prior to chemotherapy of a patient and this was overruled by the court because it had been recommended by NICE.

Limitations to Patient and Public Inclusiveness

Despite the legal and policy framework in favour of a person-centred approach, there are a number of obstacles to true inclusion of patients and the public in healthcare delivery. In particular, if we consider patient complaints and testimonials, which should be used to improve healthcare provision, it is possible to identify three types of obstacles. The first is the reliability of the data itself, the second is the ability to aggregate such information to improve healthcare provision nationwide and the third is related to flaws in the complaints system.

National surveys are not necessarily sufficiently adapted to the local situation or local needs. Researchers Wright et al. carried out a study to assess whether such performance evaluations through questionnaires were reliable (Wright et al., 2012). The conclusions of their study showed that while such evaluations may give formative feedback on a doctor's professional practice, because of the subjective nature of the feedback, such surveys should not be used in isolation. Moreover, it depends how the questions are formulated. It has been found that responses to closed-ended questions usually give positive answers about care whereas open-ended questions tend to give negative results. This is known as the 'leniency effect' (The Health Foundation, 2013). The problem with open access websites is that it is difficult to verify and check the validity of the stories and responses. Some closed access systems also exist and in these systems the patients are sent an invitation to share their care experience, but they must register to share their stories, so such systems might be more reliable.

The problem with using complaints and/or testimonials to improve the system overall is that patient complaints are not necessarily a systematic sign of failure. The other issue is that they are often emotive and specific to individual healthcare professionals. Patients might complain without taking into account wider pressures (staff workloads for example) meaning that they are unable to analyse other factors influencing the provision of healthcare. When things go wrong, the response is often to identify an individual or individuals to blame. But while individual healthcare workers should be called to account for their actions, in a large number of cases the failures stretch beyond the individuals to the system at large. In separate studies, Allsop (1994) and Lloyd-Bostock and Mulcahy (1994) underline the essential difficulties of using narratives to drive change in healthcare provision. They note that such accounts contain quite a lot of personal information which might not be relevant to, or comparable with, other cases. They underline that the strength of the emotions may not actually communicate relevant grievances. When a loved one has suffered from a serious illness, carers and family tend to look for someone to blame.

Moreover, there is no systematic nationwide policy in place or standard measure to collect people's experience of healthcare in the NHS. The methodologies used to aggregate patients' complaints are often inconsistent or do not aggregate data sufficiently to give optimal depth to complaints. Data thus remains at a raw and experimental level, non-standardised and difficult to compare. Collection of data for primary care is considered to be even more inconsistent. So, while there would seem to be a move towards giving patients opportunities to complain and seek redress, there are limits to the processing and effective use of such material.

In terms of criticisms of the complaints procedure, an investigation led by Dame Janet Smith in the Fifth Report of the Shipman Inquiry, and published in 2004, found that complaints were not always investigated properly, adequate explanations were not given, there was a failure to take account of the inherent imbalance of power between healthcare professionals and patients and there was sometimes patients' fear of retribution if they spoke up (Department of Health, 2013). There was also a certain lack of impartiality in organisations investigating their own conduct, and a lack of accountability. The charity Mencap found for example that when a death or serious incident occurs, complaints are investigated by members of staff working within the same trust or CCG where the incident occurred. Investigators might even be from the same unit or specialty (Mencap, 2007). This represents a serious conflict of interest and impartiality in the investigation. The Wilson committee also underlined some inherent difficulties for complainants using the NHS complaints procedures. First, complainants find it difficult to make their views known, but they often fail to receive a correct response (The Health Foundation, 2013).

The charity Mencap emphasised that the complaints process is slow, bureaucratic and defensive. Not only do families have to wait years to obtain justice for death caused by mistreatment or negligence, but the NHS does not seem to learn from failures and take steps to avoid such deaths or serious incidents in the future (Department of Health, 2013). The charity MIND discovered that patients find it hard to identify to whom they should complain and other inherent difficulties in navigating the complaints systems (Department of Health, 2013). This results in a high number of families not filing for redress. Healthwatch England describes the complaints system as "off-putting, complex and slow" (Healthwatch England, 2015). Mulcahy and Tritter's 1993 study of 1,640 households found that 60% of those who were dissatisfied with health services did not lodge a serious complaint because of the lack of knowledge of the complaints system, low expectations, feelings of gratitude, fear of retribution, deference to health professionals or life events. When complaints are made it is often hard for them to be followed up. Patients and families complain about a lack of responses or follow up to phone calls, impersonal letters of reply, not being kept informed of progress, inadequate replies, the length of time taken to reply (Allsop & Mulcahy, 1994). Mulcahy and Tritter also reported that people often complain about the complaints procedure because of incomplete explanations, dismissive letters, 'pseudo-apologies', technical language and defensive responses (Mulcahy & Tritter, 1993). Allsop and Mulcaly, in their analysis of patients' complaints, found that little attempt was made to translate technical or defensive material into simpler language (Allsop & Mucaly, 1994).

So while data is collected, there is no systematic or reliable way of identifying lapses in standards of care, analysing them and learning from mistakes in order to introduce change. Indeed, a Department of Health report found that while individuals may learn from change, there is no apparent collective learning process in the NHS (Department of Health, 2000). The inability to learn from incidents can be explained by a number of institutional causes: rigidity of belief, values, lack of corporate responsibility, ineffective communication, a tendency for scapegoating and difficulties in understanding complex events (Department of Health, 2000).

To sum up, the key problems identified in using patient views and complaints to improve the quality of services provision include the lack of consensus on what to report, an absence of proper linkages between reporting systems, inability to make the best use of available information, lack of analysis across different systems and inability to apply recommendations across the board. Both testimonials on care and complaints lodged by patients have the potential to drive change but the system is currently difficult to put in place.

Finally, while initiatives to include the patient and public do represent a clear shift in governance, from a top-down approach to a more inclusive approach, some argue that a person-centred health approach is also seen as being part and parcel of the post-New Public Management (NPM) public policy framework. The views of the citizen are taken into consideration in the healthcare process, but he or she also has more individual responsibilities, to take care of his/her own health and social care. The individual is thus responsible for the healthcare process by taking responsible actions to ensure that the treatment will work, by for example monitoring their weight, giving up smoking, reducing drinking, eating more healthily and taking exercise. Healthcare workers strongly encourage the individual to take care of his or her health as part of this framework. Such a rationale began essentially in 1997 with the arrival of the New Labour government and has been continued, based on the notion of agency, autonomy and self-responsibility as part of the 'responsible citizen'. Policy papers make this quite clear:

Please recognise that you can make a significant contribution to your own, and your family's, good health and wellbeing, and take personal responsibility for it (Department of Health and Social Care, Patients and the Public, 2015).

We shall set out our vision (…) to enable people to have greater control over their care and support so they can enjoy maximum independence and responsibility for their own lives (Department of Health, 2010, p. 10).

According to Pollock (2004), making an individual responsible is also a way of rationing healthcare. For example, some surgeons will decline to perform elective surgery if patients do not follow advice such as stopping smoking and losing weight. However, it is also an essential move away from a collective notion of citizenship to a more individualistic stance. The essential problem with a person-centred approach is that while life-style and individual choices may be responsible to some extent for good health, there are other more significant external factors which come into play and notably the environment and social background in which people live.

In light of the aforementioned challenges related to person and public inclusiveness, the following two case studies illustrate the importance of person-centredness in healthcare delivery, but also the current failures to integrate this approach in many NHS institutions. The first case looks at the challenges to providing true person-centred care using the negligence case in Stafford hospital as an example. The second case draws on primary evidence to illustrate the difficulties in obtaining the essential person-centred care required for a patient suffering from Parkinson's disease.

The Mid-Staffordshire Hospital Trust Scandal

The Mid-Staffordshire Hospital trust crisis is an example of why it is important to use patients' surveys, testimonials and complaints to detect failures in care and remedy them, but also the difficulties in processing complaints effectively. The specific example of Stafford Hospital is very telling because it is an appalling tale of negligence in the provision of NHS hospital care and an illustration of why current care evaluation systems are not necessarily the most effective way of assessing quality of care in NHS institutions. It also underlines the essential role that patients' complaints and stories can and should play in driving up the quality of care in the NHS. Sub-standard levels of care were uncovered at Stafford Hospital:

(…) mainly because of the persistent complaints made by a very determined group of patients and those close to them (Francis, 2013, Executive summary, p.7).

From 2009 to 2013, a total of five investigations and official reports were published, the most conclusive and complete being a final report written in 2013, as a result of a full public inquiry by Sir Robert Francis QC. The scandal came to light when the Healthcare Commission, which compiles mortality rates, became aware of an unusually high number of deaths at Stafford Hospital. While the Healthcare Commission already had concerns about the hospital at this point, the investigation was triggered when Cure the NHS, an association of relatives and patients who had experienced sub-standard levels of care at Stafford Hospital (leading to deaths in some cases), contacted the Healthcare Commission with their concerns and were asked to write a report (Healthcare Commission, 2009).

The Commission then carried out an investigation between March and October 2008 interviewing almost 300 people, including 100 patients. The Commission announced that they were leading an investigation and 103 patients and families spontaneously contacted this organisation. Within this group, 99 were critical of healthcare provided or had an experience of poor care at Stafford Hospital. The Healthcare Commission's annual survey of inpatients also showed that the trust was in the bottom 20% for performance for 39 out of 62 criteria. The reasons given for these failures were numerous. The Healthcare Commission reported that the foundation trust had not set up an effective system to admit and manage patients or monitor outcomes. The hospital trust's board and senior leaders did not acknowledge the high rates of mortality and concluded that it was due to data problems or errors. Failures to diagnose and treat patients in A&E, inadequate staffing levels and inexperienced staff were also reported (Cure the NHS, 2018).

The Healthcare Commission report was then followed by an independent inquiry led by Robert Francis QC, a barrister who had led many clinical negligence claims in the past. The results of the first public inquiry were published in 2010 and compiled evidence from over 900 families (Francis, 2010). This report focused on failings in the trust itself. It reported very basic elements of neglect in the provision of hospital care: patients not washed for up to a month, food and drink placed out of patients' reach, family members having to make sure that they arrived at meal times to feed them, neglected hygiene, etc. Families removed used bandages and dressings from public areas and cleaned the toilets themselves because they were in such a dreadful state. Patients were left for hours in soiled sheeting or forgotten on commodes. Misdiagnosis was also common during the period 2005 to 2008 and patients went for hours without food, drink or medication, inexperienced doctors were left on their own on night shifts and receptionists with no medical experience manned the A&E desk (Francis, 2010).

Numerous testimonials provided evidence of sub-standard levels of care in the hospital such as the following:

Family Account of a 96-Year-Old Patient

We got there about 10'o'clock and I couldn't believe my eyes. The door was wide open. There were people walking past. Mum was in bed with the cot sides up and she hadn't got a stitch of clothes on. I mean, she would have been horrified. She was completely naked and if I said covered in faeces, she was. It was everywhere. It was in her hair, her eyes, her nails, her hands and on all the cot side, so she had obviously been trying to lift herself up or move about, because the bed was covered and it was literally everywhere and it was dried. It would have been there a long time, it wasn't new (…) so many people must have walked past and seen her; why didn't somebody go in to her? (Francis, 2010, p. 55)

The first public inquiry of July 2010 also investigated why traditional measures of health provision had failed to detect such poor care provision. Indeed, none of the national and local institutions: the local Strategic Health Authority, the local Primary Care Trust, Monitor (the Independent Regulator of NHS Foundation trusts) and the Care Quality Commission had detected failures in the quality of care. Many of these bodies had been set up under the New Labour government to better detect failures of care.

Members of the local campaign group Cure the NHS then called for a public inquiry to understand failings in the broader context of the NHS and to avoid a repeat of such incidents in other NHS trusts. They complained that the independent inquiry published in 2010 was neither wide enough in scope nor transparent (Calkin, 2013). A full public inquiry was launched in 2010 and published in 2013.

The final 2013 report revealed that there was a chronic shortage of staff, especially nursing staff, and morale was so low that some showed a lack of compassion towards patients. Staff who wished to report the conditions were deterred from doing so because of bullying. The Francis report found that the reason behind the understaffing and lack of essential equipment on the wards was that there had been staff cuts in the 2006-7 period to try to make savings of £10m in order for the hospital to gain Foundation Trust status. Indeed, at that time the granting of Foundation Trust status gave a hospital more autonomy to run as an independent corporation, accountable to local communities rather than the central government. It also meant more budget flexibility:

This failure was in part the consequence of allowing a focus on reaching national access targets, achieving financial balance and seeking foundation trust status at the cost of delivering acceptable standards of care (Francis report, 2013, Executive summary, p. 3).

Sir Robert however underlined that much of the blame should be placed on the trust's ruling board. The action taken to investigate and try to resolve concerns was inadequate and lacked a sense of urgency. This is where the importance of patients' complaints and patient and family testimonials on care play a major role. The various quality control reports from outside bodies including the Mid-Staffordshire Healthcare Commission had given the hospital 'good' ratings. However, the trust's ruling board failed to take into account the patients' and families' complaints and a number of testimonials compiled by the hospital according to national requirements. In addition, 64 people wrote letters of complaint to the Department of Health about sub-standard care at the hospital trust between August 2005 and March 2009, but department officials failed to investigate complaints (Dominiczak & Mason, 2013). Francis also underlined that staff who tried to raise concerns were not listened to and/or bullied into leaving their jobs. For example, a staff nurse at Stafford Hospital who reported a complaint about waiting times was bullied. The trust refused to take the complaint seriously and the Royal College of Nursing advised her to 'keep her head down' (Francis, 2013). Other external reports should also have been taken into account. In 2004, the trust was re-rated by the Commission for Health Improvement as a zero-star trust and a

2007 Royal College of Surgeons report described the surgical department as 'dysfunctional'.

Both of Francis' reports were particularly critical of the failure of senior figures at the hospital and external health quality monitoring bodies to collate, analyse and take patients' complaints into consideration. Francis thus recommended, among other things, that the evaluation system be improved:

Develop and share ever improving means of measuring and understanding the performance of individual professionals, teams, units and provider organisations for the patients, the public, and all other stakeholders in the system (Francis, 2013, Executive summary, p.5)

The final 2013 report focused on investigating why the system of national inspection had failed. Francis underlined how important it was to take patients' and families' grievances into account:

This was a failure of the trust first and foremost, but it was also a national failure of the regulatory and supervisory system, which should have secured the quality and safety of patient care. Why did it have to take a determined group of families to expose those failings and campaign tirelessly for answers? (Francis, 2013, Executive summary, p. 9).

It points to why ultimately more needs to be done to use patients' complaints and stories effectively in a more coherent way. The second case study also gives support to the need to shore up the patient-centred approach, but this time beyond the hospital setting.

The Person-Centred Approach and Parkinson's Disease

This case study focuses on a family's struggle to access a joined-up package of care for a family member suffering from Parkinson's disease in a primary care setting. It illustrates how much more needs to be done to ensure that the patient and families are actually, rather than rhetorically, put at the centre of healthcare provision. Through this testimonial, it will become clear that a joined-up approach involving the patient is problematic because of the competing priorities of health and social care practitioners.

Michael[1] was diagnosed with Parkinson's on his 48th birthday. Parkinson's disease is a neurodegenerative disorder that predominately affects dopamine-producing (dopaminergic) neurons in a specific area of the brain. The progression of symptoms is often different from one person to another due to the diversity of the disease, but symptoms often include: tremor, mainly at rest and described as pill rolling tremor in hands, bradykinesia (movement disorder), limb rigidity, gait and balance problems. There is no cure and the causes are unknown but treatment options vary and include medication and surgery. While Parkinson's itself is not fatal, disease complications can be serious and lead to premature death. About one in 30 people in the UK can expect to develop this chronic illness in their lifetime. The onset of the disease is usually after 60 years old and predominantly among men (40% more men are diagnosed with Parkinson's) (Parkinson's Foundation, 2018).

Before the onset of the disease, Michael had always been very active. A keen football player, he had participated several times in the Bogle Stroll (an annual 50 km walk organised by the university during rag week), and he often cycled 15 km into the city where he worked as a Senior Lecturer at the university. But Parkinson's disease is a devastating illness and little by little Michael was forced to give up many of his favourite activities. However, he and his wife had anticipated this decline and travelled all round the world from the moment he was diagnosed to his last trip to Paris in January 2015. But the illness does not just affect the patient but also the family and especially the carer: his wife, Margaret. While Michael managed his medication and was fairly independent at the beginning, in 2009 he became confused and took an overdose of regular medication, which led to a fairly lengthy spell in hospital. From that moment on, Margaret had to be more vigilant as Michael needed more and more help with daily chores. As the disease progressed, Michael's speech also deteriorated quite significantly but at the same time Margaret also started to lose her hearing.

After a significant number of falls, the local hospital decided to place Michael in a Residential Home for respite close to the family's home. However, a month later he was reassessed as needing 24-hour nursing care and transferred to another home which could provide this care. What is important to note here is that the hospital placed Michael at an expensive home, because of the pressure to get him out of hospital and into a community setting as soon as possible. This was a turning point in his care and triggered a whole number of problems, even if it relieved Margaret of many of the pressures of sole carer at home. Indeed, she had looked after Michael with very little assistance or home help until that point.

The local hospital was covering all expenses until a decision was made about who would finance Michael's care at the home. In November 2015, after a rather gruelling process: completion of a lengthy self-assessment report for Michael and participation in a 4-hour multidisciplinary meeting (MDT) which Michael himself attended along with Margaret and one of their daughters, he was judged eligible for Continuing Healthcare (CHC) funding. CHC[2] is a package of care provided outside the hospital and funded by the NHS for individuals with significant health needs. It is unique to the British system and is only provided when a significant health need has been identified. It amounts to providing care free of charge for chronically ill patients in their own home or in a care home with all expenses covered by the NHS (Department of Health, 2012, 2018).

The multidisciplinary team, which came together to assess the patient, concluded that Michael should be eligible for CHC:

Michael has some cognitive decline, physical health frailty and behavioural issues which require frequent care provision from registered nurses and skilled carers under the management and monitoring of trained nurses.

Michael requires continuity of care provided by staff that are familiar with him and over a 24-hour basis. He requires frequent care provision and access to NHS health professionals to support his deteriorating condition.

Michael does present with complex healthcare issues which in combination interact in such a manner as to make care delivery problematic, difficult to address and require frequent changes to care planning to address care needs as they arise.

He requires support with psychological wellbeing due to loss of dignity and control of his life, experiences of hallucinations and associated anxiety. (CHC Management Report of November 2015)

This was a positive outcome for Michael because the care and attention he was receiving from nurses and care assistants at the home was excellent.

However, it became increasingly clear that the local CCG was not happy to cover the expenses of the placement. In February 2016, without properly informing the family, CCG staff decided to try and move him to cheaper accommodation. The result was a rapid deterioration in Michael's health and stress and strain for Margaret and the family. This warranted a lengthy procedure of complaint which Margaret initiated.

Margaret filed a complaint locally, not only regarding the attempt to move Michael such a long period after he had been placed at the nursing home, but also because of the way that the attempt to move him had been processed. Indeed, her letter underlined how action taken by the CCG went against the five key ingredients of patient-centred care. A lack of information and communication was experienced as the CCG began to take action without consulting the patient or family. It also violated the mutual participation and planning of a change to Michael's care package as the following letter made clear:

Dear Ms L.

Re: Continuing Healthcare Review Panel decision of 6 June 2016 in respect of Michael Hamilton.

Further to the above CHC review panel decision to recommend the transfer of my husband Michael Hamilton from Sunshine Care Home in Brisildon, where he has lived since August 2015, to a less expensive care home, I wish to appeal against this decision and to make a formal complaint about the way this matter has been dealt with by the local CCG.

My husband has suffered from Parkinson's disease for 24 years. Last August, after multiple falls, he was transferred from Capeside Hospital to Sunshine residential home for respite. A month later he was reassessed as needing 24 hour nursing care and he was transferred to Sunshine nursing home. In November he was judged eligible for Continuing Healthcare funding.

Michael has now been at Sunshine nursing home for nine months and is very well looked after. After several weeks he settled in well but unfortunately the situation has deteriorated since February following an unannounced visit from the manager of Crofton Care Home in order to assess Michael for transfer to this home. Michael found this visit, and a subsequent visit from the local CCG, extremely stressful, as his condition means that he copes very badly with any change to his circumstances. Contrary to the Health and Social Care Fundamental Standards and the CCG's own Choice and Equity policy, I was not involved in these decisions and not invited to support my husband during either visit. Michael's condition has deteriorated since these visits, to the extent that his mobility is severely compromised and he now requires a wheelchair.

We have now been told that my husband must move from Sunshine nursing home as it is too expensive, unless we can top-up the fees [topping-up fees for recipients of CHC is actually illegal], which seems more than unreasonable in the circumstances and is not sustainable long term, should he recover some of his former level of health. He is not in a fit condition to be moved, but this does not seem to be fully appreciated by the local CCG.

As requested by Ms L., I have discussed my husband's fees with the manager of Sunshine nursing home, but no variation to the current fees is possible. (Copy of Original letter, names of people and places changed)

The letter went on to list a series of grounds for complaint including the lack of information of the process to move him, the lack of compassion and sympathy shown for the strain on Michael. Margaret underlined that: "since the highly insensitive visit from the manager of Crofton House and the CCG's meeting with my husband which compounded matters, his stress levels have escalated dangerously; he is now extremely unwell and in receipt of palliative care" (Quote from original letter).

Following Margaret's appeal and a supportive letter from Michael's Consultant in Palliative Medicine, the case was put to the Continuing Healthcare Review panel. In light of firm evidence communicated to the CCG by the Consultant in Palliative Medicine and the nursing home, it was upheld that a move would pose a severe and likely risk of life-threatening consequences for Michael, so the panel decided that he would not be moved. The person-centred rights were thus upheld and the patient-centred complaints procedure successful.

A follow-up review found Michael eligible to continue to receive CHC. However, the clinical lead made it clear that she would make every attempt to reduce the amount the CCG was paying the care home. However, it transpired later that she was unable to do so.

In September 2017, a nurse reviewed Michael's case and after interviewing Margaret at length, she then had a very short meeting with Michael. A few days later, she sent a formal letter in which she claimed that Michael's situation required a completely new evaluation process and therefore a MDT would take place. The reason given for this decision was that there had been a change in his situation. There was a whole new team at the CCG and they did not seem to have taken account of the former decisions taken by the old team.

It led to a new round of stress and strain for Margaret and Michael. Margaret thus wrote yet another letter to find out why it was necessary to have a completely new evaluation of Michael's eligibility since his condition had actually deteriorated since the last review. She received no explanation, just a standard letter stating that 'due process' was being followed. Margaret wrote yet another letter to the evaluator:

Dear Ms G.,

In reply to your letter of 22 September 2017, you have not addressed any of my concerns. I do not accept that in this case due process is being followed in accordance with the National Framework for NHS CHC and NHS funded nursing care, November 2012 (revised). Practice Guidance notes in paragraph PG 67 state that: "A DST will not be required where:- the person has previously had a positive checklist and full DST completed by an MDT and there has been no material change in their needs ".

My husband's care needs were clearly stated in 2015: "continuity of care provided by staff that are familiar with him over a 24-hour basis." He requires "frequent care provision and access to NHS health professionals to support his deteriorating condition". Since then, he now needs more care, for example, at times requiring 2 people to move him to the toilet and to a wheelchair when he is unable to use his rollator.

As you claim that your review identified a need to go back to the CHC process, I would be grateful if you could forward to me a copy of your annotations of the original DST considered by the panel on 10 November 2015, so that I can see how you may have considered that my husband's condition has improved since then. (You were informed by a senior nurse at Sunshine care home that it has deteriorated.)

My previous complaint of 2016 to the local CCG regarding the lack of consultation was upheld. The recurrence of this same fault in this annual review goes against the CCG's stated undertaking to rectify their processes. (See also paragraph 67.2 in the Framework regarding consultation).

I shall be away from 28 September to 11 October and it is imperative that you do not contact my husband in any way during my absence, as any suggestion of a change in his circumstances is extremely stressful for him, and therefore very harmful to his health, and contrary to the person-centred approach required by the CHC National Framework. (Copy of original letter sent to CCG in September 2017)

From September to November, Margaret was in a particularly bad state at the thought of going through a further process. On 23 September, she sent an e-mail to her younger daughter:

Had another letter just saying the same as before and not answering any of my points. Am so fed up. I don't know what it will do to your dad if we have to go through that whole process again. (Copy of original e-mail sent to daughter)

Margaret was disconcerted by the failure of the CCG to communicate and explain the purpose of the new DST and the lack of regard for the previous failures in the communication of possible changes to Michael's care package. Perhaps the reason that it had been so easy to overturn the 2015 and 2016 decisions and request a whole new MDT was because the whole CHC process is very subjective in nature. In fact, the National Guidance Framework is, in some ways, at odds with legal precedents by which it claims to abide, and especially the Coughlan Case.

The Coughlan Case was a legal case setting a precedent to distinguish when someone's healthcare needs are no longer the responsibility of the local authorities and should therefore be paid for by the NHS. The Court of Appeal said, "If the nursing services are (i) merely incidental or ancillary to the provision of the accommodation which a local authority is under a duty to provide…and (ii) of a nature which it can be expected that an authority whose primary responsibility is to provide social services can be expected to provide, then they can be provided [by the local authority]." (R. v. North and East Devon Health Authority, ex parte Coughlan [1999] EWCA Civ 1871, [2001] Q.B. 213 at 239, para. 53, Court of Appeal (England and Wales)). In fact, on the basis of such legal precedence, the majority of patients receiving care in nursing home should be eligible for CHC.

By reading a number of narratives on a special dedicated website (Care to be Different), the family realised that Michael's original allocation and subsequent maintenance of CHC could be easily overturned. Indeed, a number of testimonials showed how CHC was often granted and then withdrawn. The argument that CHC staff put forward is that if the patient stabilises, i.e. his or her situation does not change (he does not improve but his health has not significantly declined from the previous review), then it might be possible to remove CHC because the illness is more manageable and/or less unpredictable.

Despite a very detailed self-assessment report which Margaret and her younger daughter wrote together on behalf of Michael, which reconfirmed that the previous assessment of Michael's state of health and needs were still at the same level and/or had actually increased, the decision was taken to remove CHC. The final assessment noted that:

There is no evidence to suggest that Michael Hamilton's day to day care needs are intensive in any way and all of his care needs are met through the provision of routine nursing care.

Michael's day to day care needs do not appear complex in any way. (CHC Management Report of November 2017)

The family decided to start an appeal against the decision because the CCG's most recent evaluation completely contradicted the previous 2015 evaluation. Moreover, the social worker on the assessment panel had never even met Michael before the MDT and the representative from the care home was the Area Care Representative, so was not particularly involved in Michael's day-to-day care. There was no input from the nursing staff who had looked after Michael on a day-to-day basis.

After the review and the outcome in November 2017, which was again very stressful and gruelling for both Margaret and Michael, Michael's health declined significantly. He developed a swallowing problem and sadly died three months later after several weeks in hospital. Although premature death is often a result of Parkinson's, the family believed that his rapid deterioration could well have been linked to the stress and strain of the CHC process.

Michael's testimonial shows a number of failures in the provision of a patient-centred approach including failure to fully inform, communicate and enable the patient and family to participate in care planning and care coordination. The problem also lies with the underlying aims of the complaints. In the case of Michael, we are dealing with different levels of care in a community setting where the boundaries of rights and imposing those rights remain rather obscure.

The Wilson committee underlined a number of difficulties for complainants using the NHS complaints procedures. First, in making their views known and also having a correct response. Indeed, in Michael's case we can note that, in the first instance, the family was satisfied with the response to Margaret's complaint but in the second case, the complaint was completely ignored. The amount of time and energy the family spent navigating the complaints procedure and understanding how they should complain against undue process was significant. This results in a high number of families not filing for redress. There may also be an obstacle of capability for many families seeking redress. Complainants must master the jargonistic language and discourse and acquire full knowledge of legislation when filing complaints. Moreover, Michael's family was also surprised by the lack of impartiality of the investigation when they started an appeal against the decision to remove CHC. The Local Resolution panel consisted of the clinical lead who chaired the original MDT meeting and the nurse who led the MDT.

When complaints are made it is often hard for them to be followed through: lack of responses or follow up to phone calls, impersonal letters of reply, not being kept informed of progress, inadequate and late replies, etc. (Allsop & Mulcahy, 1994). All these were evident in Michael's story. In summary, in Michael's case, many of the quality dimensions of person-centred care were not in place. Indeed, the CHC team did not pay attention to his physical and environmental needs when trying to move him. Empathy and respect were often lacking during Margaret's communication with the CHC team and a continuity of care or smooth transitions did not appear to be the key priorities of the care providers at the CCG. Findings from a National Voices report (2017) suggests that personalised care planning in the NHS remains very uneven and largely absent in many NHS settings. The same report concluded that family involvement also remains marginal to the practice of person-centred care.

CONCLUSION

While the new clinical governance framework has provided impetus for person-inclusiveness, in practice the implementation of legislation and policy recommendations is fraught with difficulties. The clinical governance framework provides for patient and public inclusiveness, but this has not prevented substandard levels of care or active patient/public exclusion in the health delivery process. One of the major difficulties in providing patient and public involvement across the UK is the very localised nature of healthcare delivery, which we will examine in the next chapter.

REFERENCES

Allsop, J. (1994). Two sides to every story: Complainants' and doctors' perspectives in disputes about medical care in a general practice setting. *Law & Policy*, *16*(2), 149–184. doi:10.1111/j.1467-9930.1994.tb00121.x

Allsop, J., & Mulcahy, L. (1994). Dealing with Clinical Complaints. *Quality in Health Care*, *4*(2), 135–143. doi:10.1136/qshc.4.2.135 PMID:10151613

Calkin, S. (2013, January 31). Ten Frequently Asked Questions: What is the Francis Report. *Nursing Times*. Retrieved January 10, 2019, from https://www.nursingtimes.net/news/reviews-and-reports/francis-report/10-frequently-asked-questions-what-is-the-francis-report/5054230.article.

Cure the NHS. (2018, December 18). *About Cure the NHS*. Retrieved November 8, 2019, from http://www.curethenhs.co.uk/about-cure-the-nhs/

Department of Health. (1999). *Supporting doctors, protecting patients*. Department of Health.

Department of Health. (2000). *An organisation with a memory: Report of an expert group on learning from adverse events in the NHS*. Stationery Office.

Department of Health. (2010). *Equity and excellence: Liberating the NHS*. HMSO.

Department of Health. (2013). *A review of the NHS hospital's complaints system: Putting patients back in the picture*. HMSO.

Department of Health. (2018). *Framework for NHS Continuing Healthcare and NHS-funded Nursing Care*. Department of Health. Retrieved April 12, 2020, from https://www.gov.uk/government/publications/national-framework-for-nhs-continuing-healthcare-and-nhs-funded-nursing-care

Department of Health and Social Care. (2015, October 14). *The NHS Constitution for England*. Retrieved on April 15, 2020, from https://www.gov.uk/government/publications/the-nhs-constitution-for-england/the-nhs-constitution-for-england#patients-and-the-public-your-rights-and-the-nhs-pledges-to-you

Dominiczak, P., & Mason, R. (2013, March 24). More than 60 Mid Staffordshire hospital complaints to Government ignored. *The Telegraph*. Retrieved January 17, 2017, from https://www.telegraph.co.uk/news/politics/9951218/More-than-60-Mid-Staffordshire-hospital-complaints-to-Government-ignored.html

England, H. (2015). *Healthwatch England annual report 2015/6: Every voice matters*. Healthwatch.

Francis, R. (2010). Robert Francis inquiry report into Mid-Staffordshire NHS Foundation Trust. HSC 1998/822. Crown.

Francis, R. (2013). *Report of the Mid-Staffordshire NHS Foundation Trust Public Inquiry*. Stationery Office. HC 947.

Guiliani, C., Gault, N., Fares, V., Jegu, J., Eleni, S., Biga, J., & Vidal-Trecan, G. (2009). Evolution of patients' complaints in a French university hospital: Is there a contribution of a law regarding patients' rights? *BMC Health Services Research*, *9*(141). Retrieved December 16, 2018, from https://bmchealthservres.biomedcentral.com/articles/10.1186/1472-6963-9-141 PMID:19660131

Ham, C. (2009). *Health policy in Britain* (6th ed.). Palgrave Macmillan. doi:10.1007/978-1-137-01397-2

Healthcare Commission. (2009). *Investigation into Mid Staffordshire NHS Trust Foundation Trust (Summary Report)*. Healthcare Commission.

Lawson, D. (2015, May 1). Explained: The legal challenges to CCG decision making. *HSJ*. Retrieved May 28, 2018, from https://www.hsj.co.uk/commissioning/explained-the-legal-challenges-to-ccg-decision-making/5084425.article

Lloyd-Bostock, S., & Mulcahy, L. (1994). The social psychology of making and responding to hospital complaints: An account model of complaint processes. *Law & Policy*, *16*(2), 123–147. doi:10.1111/j.1467-9930.1994.tb00120.x

Mead, N., & Bower, P. (2000). Patient-centredness: A conceptual framework and review of the empirical literature. *Social Science & Medicine*, *51*(7), 1087–1110. doi:10.1016/S0277-9536(00)00098-8 PMID:11005395

Medical Workforce Unit of the Royal College of Physicians London. (2019). *Focus on physicians: Census of consultant physicians and higher specialty trainees 2018*. Royal College of Physicians, Royal College of Physicians of Edinburgh and the Royal College of Physicians and Surgeons of Glasgow. Retrieved March 28, 2020, from https://www.rcplondon.ac.uk/projects/outputs/focus-physicians-2018-19-census-uk-consultants-and-higher-specialty-trainees

Mencap. (2007). *Death by indifference*. Mencap.

Mulcahy, L., & Tritter, J. (1993). *Dissatisfaction, grievances and complaints in the NHS, A report to the Department of Health*. HMSO.

National Voices. (2017). *Person-centred care in 2017. Evidence from service users*. National Voices.

NHS England. (2017). *Patient and public participation policy*. NHS England. Retrieved March 10, 2018, from https://www.england.nhs.uk/wp-content/uploads/2017/04/ppp-policy.pdf

Parkinson's Foundation. (2018). *What is Parkinson's?* Parkinson's Foundation. Retrieved June 18, 2019, from https://www.parkinson.org/understanding-parkinsons/what-is-parkinsons

Pollock, A. M. (2004). *NHS plc: The privatisation of our healthcare*. Verso.

Reader, T., Gillespie, A., & Roberts, J. (2013). Patient complaints in healthcare systems: A systematic review and coding taxonomy. *BMJ Journals*, *23*(8), 678–689. PMID:24876289

Resolution, N. H. S. (2018, July 12). *NHS Resolution presses ahead with mediation as litigation decreases but claims costs continue to rise*. Retrieved on April 12, 2020, from https://resolution.nhs.uk/2018/07/12/nhs-resolution-presses-ahead-with-mediation-as-litigation-decreases-but-claims-costs-continue-to-rise/

Rogers, C. R. (1951). *Client-centred therapy: Its current practice, implications and theory*. Houghton Mifflin.

Starfield, B. (2011). Is patient-centered care the same as person-focused care? *The Permanente Journal*, *15*(2), 63–69. doi:10.7812/TPP/10-148 PMID:21841928

The Health Foundation. (2013). *Measuring patient experience*. The Health Foundation.

WHO. (2007, November 25). People-centred health care. In *International symposium on people-centred healthcare: Reorienting health systems in the 21st Century*. The Tokyo International Forum. Retrieved March 13, 2018, from https://apps.who.int/iris/bitstream/handle/10665/207004/9789290613930_eng.pdf;jsessionid=44177C8B98F1EA1C95E4857B98F23663?sequence=1

Wright, C., Richards, S. H., Hill, J., Roberts, J., Norman, G. R., Greco, M., Taylor, M. R. S., & Campbell, J. L. (2012). Multisource feedback in evaluating the performance of doctors: The example of the UK General Medical Council patient and colleague questionnaires. *Academic Medicine*, *87*(12), 1668–1678. doi:10.1097/ACM.0b013e3182724cc0 PMID:23095930

ENDNOTES

1 The names of people and places have been changed for legal reasons.

2 For a more in depth study of CHC, please refer to the case study in Chapter 6

Chapter 5
The Place-Based Challenge

ABSTRACT

When considering the provision of healthcare services, it is necessary to examine action at a local level and problems that local health service providers must face. This is essentially because it is within individual communities and neighbourhoods that most public healthcare interventions take place. Local intervention is also important in order to coordinate a more even pattern of healthcare provision across the regions. There are significant disparities between regions and inter-regions of the UK. Recent cuts to public services, welfare benefits, and public employment have severely affected those regions. This chapter will thus explore health inequalities and inequity of supply across the devolved administrations, regions, and sub-regions. It will then review policy to address health inequalities and consider to what extent the current public health service governance framework, and especially health service provision at the local level, can mitigate disparities in health outcomes. It includes a short section on the response to the Covid-19 pandemic in the regions.

INTRODUCTION

Governance issues and conflicts in terms of how to deal with health issues are evident if we look at the local dimension of healthcare delivery. The United Kingdom has a very specific situation in that local government and local authorities, who are in part responsible for healthcare delivery, do not have any codified rules or any constitutional guarantees. National parliament is

DOI: 10.4018/978-1-7998-3928-6.ch005

sovereign and therefore NHS institutions, while they collaborate with local authorities and social services in the delivery of healthcare, are actually accountable to central government. The absence of constitutional checks and balances in the British system of government means that new legislation may be implemented and both local government and NHS institutions need to adapt service delivery to such regulations. A lack of information and ability to follow such evolving legislation is a major issue for National Health Service (NHS) providers in the localities (European Observatory on Health Systems and Policies, 2015).

The situation has become even more complex since the move towards devolving responsibility for the delivery of healthcare. From 1997 onwards and the process of devolution, which transferred powers to manage health to separate bodies in Scotland, Wales, Northern Ireland and England, the nations of the UK began to manage healthcare quite differently. Health services are funded via block grants for Scotland, Wales and Northern Ireland and a budget is allocated to England from the UK government. Each health department then funds health organisations in the regions and sub-regions of the separate nations who arrange services on behalf of their patients (European Observatory on Health Systems and Policies, 2015). Further transfer of power to the local level was also encouraged by New Labour and set out in the publication *Shifting the Balance of Power: The Next Steps* (Department of Health, 2001). Whereas healthcare delivery used to be divided quite distinctly between on the one hand, strategy, policy and management, and on the other hand, medical and clinical care, the move to a more decentralised system of healthcare has resulted in a blurring of the two divisions (Grosios, Gahan, & Burbidge, 2010).

When considering the provision of healthcare services in a country, it is necessary to examine action at a local level and problems that local health service providers must face. This is essentially because it is within individual communities and neighbourhoods that most public health interventions take place. Local intervention is also important in order to co-ordinate a more even pattern of healthcare provision across the regions. Where regions or localities are seen to be failing in their provision of good quality services, action is needed at both the local and national level. This is because the NHS is a national institution and should therefore provide for the needs of all its citizens in an equitable way. The role of healthcare services in the region goes beyond the sole domain of health. Quality healthcare can contribute to attracting new industries and skilled people, and is important for the social and economic prosperity of the region. Health service providers also contribute to the overall economy of a region, raising both GDP and employment levels, with clear linkages and multiplier effects. Issues such as coping with an ageing population, poor health and higher expectations for healthcare delivery are ever more evident at the local level and raise even more governance challenges since health performance is so uneven in the United Kingdom.

It has become clear over recent decades that there are significant disparities between regions and inter-regions. When looking at a wide set of indicators in the regions[1], there is a definite north-south divide in terms of health. Sub-regional disparities are often even greater than those between regions, but this does not diminish the weight of data that shows that the majority of southern regions fare much better than their northern[2] counterparts for health outcomes. In England in particular, recent cuts to public services, welfare benefits and public jobs have severely affected those regions. Overall, health inequalities have risen. Life expectancy has increased steadily in the United Kingdom, but some areas are experiencing declining life expectancy once again. This chapter will thus explore local governance policy. It will then review uneven health performance across the regions and policies to address such health inequalities. It will consider how England and each of the devolved administration is performing and to what extent the current public health service governance framework, and especially NHS health service provision, at the local level can mitigate disparities in health outcomes.

REGIONAL HEALTH POLICY: A RETURN TO LOCALISM FOR HEALTH PROVISION?

From 1998, with the arrival of New Labour in government and the subsequent devolution process, emphasis was put on the need for local action for health. This drive towards decentralisation has been continued and reinforced. Yet the recent focus on driving improvements in the provision of health services through local governance is not a new phenomenon, but actually a leap back to the past when health provision was indeed completely dependent on local providers, before the NHS was created in 1948[3]. Emphasis on localism or 'new localism' was the mantra of the New Labour government and such an approach has gradually changed the nature of public healthcare provision today. Localism implies first and foremost the devolution or, at the very least, the decentralisation of powers to local bodies in order to give local managers and stakeholders the powers to implement national strategies, but also to better meet the needs of the population. However, the central steer still comes or should come from central government and this is the essential difference between 'new localism' and 'old localism'. In addition, another major difference between former and current localism is that power has not just been devolved to the local government, as was the case with old localism, but to a range of local stakeholders or governors in public services including NHS health providers.

Aneurin Bevan, the founder of the NHS, argued that it was important to provide strong central management of NHS services because local government service provision was far too uneven. Indeed, Bevan expressed concern that devolved power would lead to spatial unevenness and especially poor performance in resource-stretched areas (Ministry of Health, 1944). While localism was disbanded on the creation of the NHS, regional governance has been significant ever since the inception of the NHS (Ham, 2009). On the creation of the NHS in 1948, regional hospital boards managed hospitals and co-ordinated services. They saw their responsibilities rise in 1974 when they became regional health authorities. In 1992, regional branches of the NHS Management Executive were set up to co-manage, with the regional health authorities, the administration of health in the regions. Under New Labour the dynamics of power were changed with the abolition of regional powers, but they were replaced by Strategic Health Authorities (SHAs) in 1992 to oversee the work of the Primary Care Trusts (PCTs) in the regions and act on behalf of the Secretary of State (Ham, 2009).

Unlike Bevan, successive governments since the late 1990s have argued that the transfer of public health from a centralised NHS to local government is important because local government provides services that are directly related to health such as housing, jobs, culture, leisure and the environment. Government policy papers have argued that it is at the local and micro level that improvements to health can be made (Department of Health, 1997). The emphasis on place in public healthcare provision gathered momentum when New Labour came into office. Devolution of powers also saw a significant rise in the responsibility of regions to manage health.

A clear devolution of powers to the regions was at the heart of New Labour's reforms in creating PCTs in England and encouraging trusts to apply for foundation trust status. As Ham underlines, these reforms were made to move from a hierarchical and central management of health to a decentralised NHS. The aim was to limit the role of the Department of Health but also the responsibility for the adverse effects of management which led to complaints from NHS staff and the public alike. PCTs were expected to take over the role of setting priorities and standards to ensure high quality service provision (Ham, 2009).

Greater decentralisation of powers to local institutions was also at the heart of the framework. As the *NHS Plan* (Department of Health, 2000) underlined, it was unthinkable for local hospitals to be run from Whitehall. Local authorities were considered to be in the best position to deal with local needs. We may also note a decentralisation of financial arrangements. Although central taxation remains the key provider of financial resources for the NHS, devolution in managing these budgets has taken place over the years. Until the introduction of the internal market in 1991, the Regional Health Authorities (answering directly to the Department of Health) were responsible for the allocation of the NHS budget to service providers. After 1991, this responsibility passed to the lower local tier, the District Health Authorities, and later to the General Practitioner (GP) fund-holding practices.

But it was in 2000 that decentralisation was truly reinforced with the NHS Service Plan, which resulted in the transfer of a number of powers from centralised NHS bodies to local structures. Hospital autonomy was also strongly encouraged. The 2003 Health and Social Care Act further strengthened the autonomy of hospitals in localities. Finally, decentralisation was pushed one step further with the Health and Social Care Act of 2012. Since then, budgeting has passed down to Clinical Commissioning Groups (CCGs) and local authorities in England.

Since 2015, English regions have also been given the opportunity to bid for full control of their health and social care budgets. In April 2016, Greater Manchester was the first English region to take control of health spending. Indeed, 10 boroughs, 15 NHS trusts and 12 CCGs are now jointly responsible for a £6 billion-a-year health and social care budget in this region. The outcomes of such policies are yet to be seen. It is unclear to what extent these policies will boost growth and health outcomes in the North because observers have noted that the budget of £28 billion is unlikely to be sufficient to tackle the complex health challenges in the region and any benefits may be offset by local authority budget cuts. Nevertheless, the role of healthcare providers remains crucial in addressing the problems of ill health in the Northern regions.

A PWC report concluded that recent reforms have resulted in a "complex middle-ground between central control, devolved decision making and a market-based approach", which is considered to be "misaligned to today's challenges, adds complexity and duplication, and frequently hinders the progress local leaders are seeking to make" (PWC, 2016, p. 1). There is also some concern that passing budgeting to the local level and independent budgeting might have resulted in an ever more unequal distribution of health funds across localities. This could happen in a system of allocation flows to decentralised units. Danny Dorling underlines that the creation of CCGs under the Health and Social Care Act of 2012 and the transfer of powers once held by the Secretary of State for Health, essentially amounts to passing the legal duty to secure comprehensive healthcare to local commissioners and providers (Dorling, 2013, p. 84). Indeed, this Act altered the original obligation of the Secretary of State to provide a comprehensive health service. Under the New Act, there is no longer a legal obligation for the Secretary of State for Health or NHS professionals to *provide* a comprehensive healthcare system even if the former has a legal duty to *promote* a comprehensive service. Indeed, Section 1 of the NHS Act states:

The Secretary of State must continue the promotion in England of a comprehensive health service designed to secure improvement—

a) *in the physical and mental health of the people of England, and*
b) *in the prevention, diagnosis and treatment of physical and mental illness (Health and Social Care Act, 2012, Section 1)*

Dorling argues that this essentially represents a move back to the former system that existed before the creation of the NHS, whereby health provision was contingent on what local charity boards and hospitals could provide and depended heavily on the affluence of the area. In addition, CCGs are not responsible for all children and adults in that area because the patient populations are selected from GPs lists[4], so CCGs provide care for a select population rather than a pre-determined geographical area, which means that some people may be excluded (Dorling, 2013). Pollock and Price (2013) also contend that the role of the Secretary of State and commissioners to provide equity of access to the population has been diminished under the new act and the reduction of the role of the secretary of state to a promoter and not a provider of healthcare:

The Secretary of State does not have a duty to promote equity of access apart from a vague duty to "have regard to the need to reduce inequalities between the people of England with respect to the benefits that they can obtain from the health service". The NHS Commissioning Board will not have a general power of direction over consortiums or be under a duty to ensure equal access for equal need to health services. A vague equity duty also applies to commissioning groups in the form of a requirement to "have regard to the need to reduce inequalities between patients".

Equality of access is not a required outcome of commissioning groups' duty to secure "continuous improvement" from the provision of services; nor is it part of annual "commissioning plans" that groups will be required to prepare. These will cover only continuous improvement and the financial duty to break even. (Pollock & Price, 2013, p. 19)

The Secretary of State for Health still maintains the overall responsibility for the business and policies of the department, including: financial control, oversight of all NHS delivery and performance, mental health and patient safety. However, the legal terminology "promoter" remains very vague and is aimed more at encouraging a universal supply of healthcare rather than taking full responsibility to provide one.

The move to localism and the transfer of health governance to local governments under the Health and Social Act of 2012 has thus reignited claims of uneven supply in line with Bevan's arguments. While public health budgets were initially ring-fenced in the local authorities, there is pressure to remove this in order to have more budget flexibility, faced with the further 10% cut to local budgets in 2015-6.

So while many of the government texts promote the advantages of managing health services at the local level, there are some essential weaknesses to the decentralisation process which have already been underlined on a global level. Indeed, after reviewing the literature on decentralisation, the United States Agency for International Development (USAID) funded Partnership for Health Reform noted a number of problems arising from this process. First, service provision may become controlled at the local level by elites who are not as responsive to the needs of the population as the government. Urban populations have significant political influence compared to rural populations and may be in a position to keep a larger share of resources. Decentralisation means that it is more difficult to control provision of services and there may be a degree of local-level corruption. Some localities may lack the managerial skills and expertise needed in the health domain. Decentralisation inevitably means smaller scale and thus less well-resourced providers to pay for training and skills of their staff, which may result in lower quality care. Smaller organisations tend to have less bargaining power and less ability to achieve economies of scale. Finally, smaller scales are said to have less scope to tackle inequalities for the population, but also for health workers

(Rannan-Eliya & Somanathan, 2006). However, transferring governance to the devolved administrations has been heralded as a success.

Local Governance in the Devolved Administrations

After devolution, Scotland and Wales decided to abandon the purchaser/provider split in 2004 and 2009 respectively, and created health boards similar to those that had existed in the 1980s. In Wales, the system of performance management in the NHS was criticised in the second Wanless Report because of a lack of incentive systems or best practice resolutions (Wanless, 2004; Bevan et al., 2014). Moreover, the Auditor General for Wales stated that the performance management arrangements had not improved performance, especially waiting times, because of lack of incentives and sanctions (Bevan et al., 2014). In 2009, the Five-Year Service, Workforce and Financial Strategic Framework for NHS Wales was introduced in Wales (NHS Wales, 2010). This transferred significant powers to the Health and Social Care Committee of the National Assembly for Wales, to seven Local Health Boards (LHBs) and to the trust chief executive governing three NHS trusts. These institutions have responsibility for planning and providing health services for the Welsh population, guided by the policy framework set forth by the Welsh Minister for Health and Social Services. Targets, checks and balances are part and parcel of the Welsh system. The Department of Health and Social Services, part of the Welsh Government, sets out objectives for the NHS and time lines for care delivery. NHS Trusts and Local Health Boards (LHBs) are responsible for meeting those targets and producing planning documents in order to achieve given objectives. Care is delivered by the LHBs according to these targets. The Welsh National Advisory Board, the All Wales Medicines Strategy Groups and the Bevan Commission give advice on the development and delivery of policy. Moreover, as in the English system, NICE gives advice to and develops quality indicators for Welsh health administrators. Health and social care delivery is implemented at a local level by the LHBs in collaboration with the Local Authorities (Single Integrated Plans). NHS Wales is monitored and regulated by Community Health Councils (CHCs) and Healthcare Inspectorate Wales (National Assembly for Wales, 2015). The performance management system in Wales is focused on two sets of core delivery targets. These are called Tier 1 targets, which are "key priorities where immediate improvement is necessary or where performance at defined target levels must be sustained" and are "subject to very close attention by

Figure 1. Structure of the NHS in Wales
Source: National Assembly for Wales (2015)

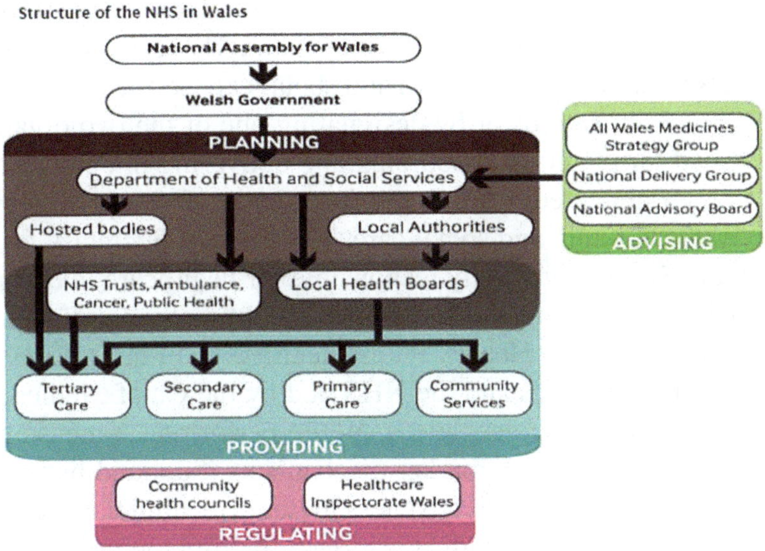

health boards, trusts and Welsh Government (through national monitoring)" (NHS Wales, 2011; Bevan et al., 2014).

In Scotland, the purchaser-provider split was considered to be ineffective because it created "perverse incentives... where 'failing' boards were 'bailed out' with extra cash and those managing their finances well were not incentivised" (Steel & Cylus, 2012; Bevan et al., 2014). There were also unfavourable reports on waiting times. Scotland therefore ushered in a system which transformed primary care in order to shift the balance away from acute care and episodic interaction to a system which gave more priority to preventive medicine, support for self-care and anticipatory medicine. As Greer (2004) underlines, after devolution England continued to intensify the role of the market in the supply of public healthcare, whereas Scotland focused on professionalism. Scotland removed the layers of hierarchy and the 'command and control' system, which effectively led to a closer relationship with the chief executives and workers on the front line. According to Dayan and Edwards (2017), Scotland's unique system "focuses on engaging the altruistic professional motivations of frontline staff to do better". The governance system in Scotland can be described as one of continuity and consistency, which is necessary for quality improvement. This is in sharp contrast to the English and Welsh systems which have experienced reorganisation after reorganisation and significant changes to governance structures. In Scotland, the Directorate for Health and Social Care is in charge of health policy, the administration of the NHS, community care and part of its remit relates to social work. The NHS in Scotland consists of 13 NHS Boards and 31 local authorities which promote integration of certain health and social care services either through the creation of Joint Boards or by designating one of the two organisations to take the lead for planning, resourcing and delivering integrated services. Funding is then allocated accordingly in order to develop strategic plans for the delivery of health and social care. The Cabinet Secretary for Health, Wellbeing and Sport is primarily responsible for healthcare in co-operation with the Minister for Public Health and the Minister for Sport, Health Improvement and Mental Health. Public health is the remit of the Scottish Executive, local authorities and the NHS, led by the Chief Medical Officer (National Assembly for Wales, 2015). While performance measures in the UK focus on alignment with market mechanisms, Scotland has developed measurements of safety and effectiveness in line with clinicians' evaluations of health performance and indicators. Health improvement, Efficiency, Access and Treatment (HEAT) targets have also been introduced, organised by a delivery group within the health department to agree to local delivery plans within each board. An outcomes framework is used to monitor the work of the Joint Boards, the NHS Boards and local authorities. In order to monitor health and social care and set goals to improve the health of the population, a Clinical Standards Board was set up in Scotland. This was followed by the establishment of NHS Quality Improvement Scotland in 2003 (which has since been renamed Healthcare Improvement Scotland). Moreover, the Scottish Patient Safety Programme was introduced and, as part of this programme, which monitors patient safety in acute, mental and primary healthcare, clinicians and managers receive training. The institution is also in charge of refining skills and methods, and overseeing changes to and provision of healthcare (Dayan and Edwards, 2017).

Northern Ireland's original performance management system was criticised for a lack of appropriate performance structures, information and clear and effective incentives (Appleby, 2005). Reforms in Northern Ireland have been slow because of the dissolution of the Assembly. Nevertheless, the Health and Social Care (Reform) Act (NI) of 2009 led to the creation of the Health and Social Care Board, which was a large commissioning body supported by five local commissioning groups across the region and five coterminous health and social care trusts to provide care (Bevan et al., 2014). Northern Ireland chose to maintain the purchaser-provider split but at the same time

Figure 2. Structure of the NHS in Scotland
Source: National Assembly for Wales (2015)

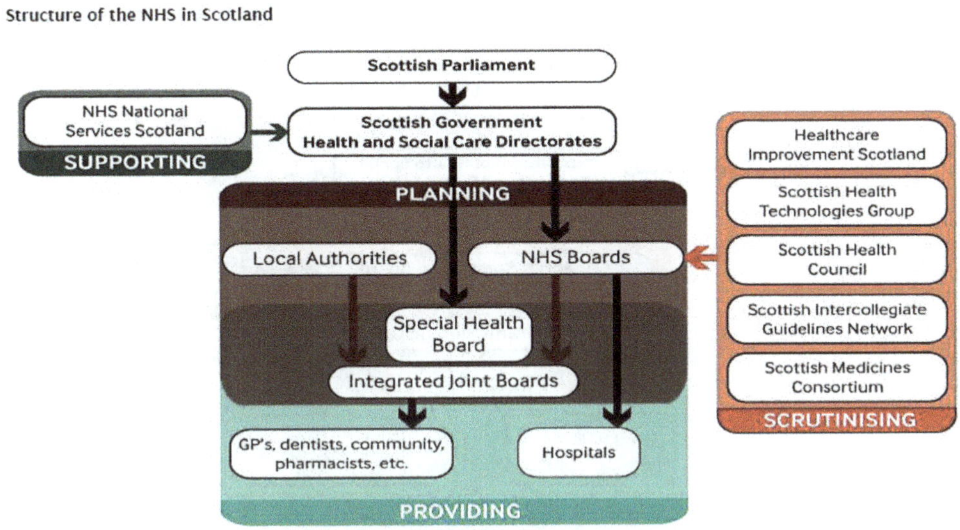

policy emphasises co-operation rather than competition which was reinforced only in England, especially following the 2012 Health and Social Care Act. The Regulation and Quality Improvement Authority (RQIA) oversees and promotes accessibility of health and social care services in Northern Ireland. NICE also advises Northern Ireland. RQIA's role is to ensure that NICE's advice is implemented (National Assembly for Wales, 2015).

Such governance arrangements have had an impact on performance in the four nations of the UK. However, before turning to specific health performance in the four countries, this next section will consider health inequities which inevitably have a significant impact on performance.

INEQUITIES AND HEALTHCARE PROVISION

A central theme in the delivery of public health services at the regional level is how to improve outcomes and fight against both inequalities and inequities in terms of health outcomes. The WHO distinguishes between inequality and inequity in the following way:

Health inequalities can be defined as differences in health status or in the distribution of health determinants between different population groups.

Figure 3. Structure of the NHS in Northern Ireland
Source: National Assembly for Wales (2015)

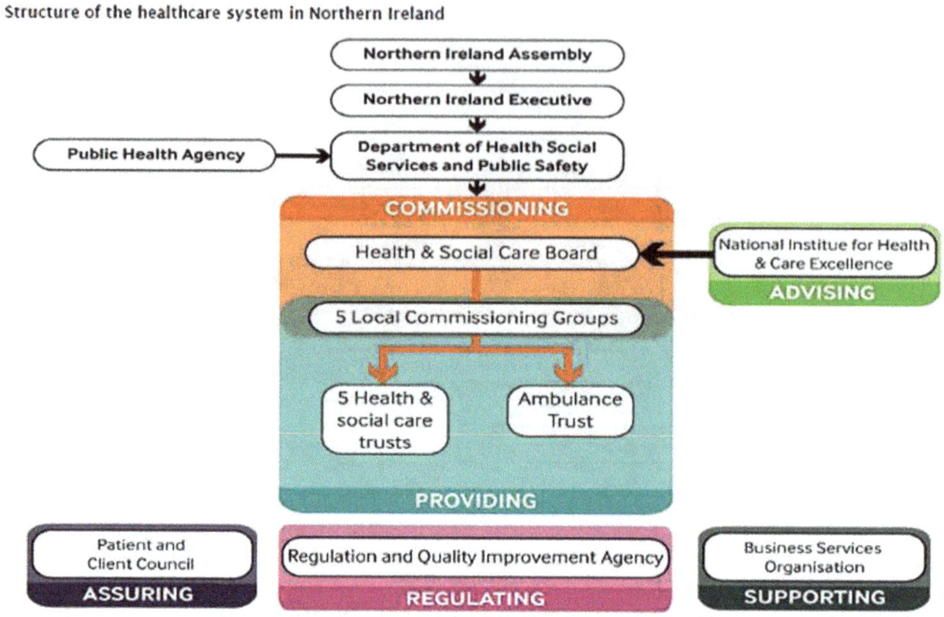

For example, differences in mobility between elderly people and younger populations or differences in mortality rates between people from different social classes. It is important to distinguish between inequality in health and inequity. Some health inequalities are attributable to biological variations or free choice and others are attributable to the external environment and conditions mainly outside the control of the individuals concerned. In the first case it may be impossible or ethically or ideologically unacceptable to change the health determinants and so the health inequalities are unavoidable. In the second, the uneven distribution may be unnecessary and avoidable as well as unjust and unfair, so that the resulting health inequalities also lead to inequity in health (WHO, 2017).

Parkin (2017) qualifies equity in a number of different ways: equal use of health services for equal needs for healthcare, equal use of health services for equal willingness to pay for that use, equal health outcomes for equal merit, equal healthcare payment by people for equal ability to pay for that healthcare, equal expenditure on people for equal health deficit. Other principles may also go against the notion of equity. Indeed, the utilitarian principle states that one should maximise society's welfare even if that means creating inequities. There is therefore a significant conflict between equity and equality principles because the conceptualisation of both notions is essentially normative, based on individual or collective value judgments.

Questions of equity involve normative responses as to whether healthcare should be financed according to ability to pay or not. Regressive systems are considered to be those whereby the proportion of income spent on health is lower for the high incomes than for low incomes. Horizontal equity involves providing healthcare in relation to needs. Horizontal inequity is said to occur when need factors are assessed and it is found that healthcare services are affected by non-need factors, i.e. when individuals with the same needs consume different amounts of care. Equity is therefore the term that is used to describe access to healthcare services. However, when distribution of healthcare is discussed, the term inequality is more frequently used. Health policy debates often centre on different levels of health according to socio-economic status. In Britain, the guiding principles of the NHS have generally been that there should be equity in supply of healthcare; equal use of health services for equal need irrespective of the ability to pay:

The NHS is a great national institution. The principles it was founded on are as important now as they were then: free at the point of use and available to everyone based on need, not ability to pay. (Department of Health, 2010, p.1).

The next two sections will reflect on these inequalities and the effectiveness of government policy to mitigate problems of poor health.

Inequalities in Health Performance in the Regions

The emergence of health inequalities in terms of poorer outcomes in certain regions can be related to the rise and fall of industry, especially in the Northern regions, but also in parts of the Midlands too. Deindustrialisation, the absolute decline of mining and heavy industry, particularly hit the northern regions hard. These regions were well known for poor health performance, but ill health continued to mark the local population even after the closure of many mines and factories from the 1960s onwards. Indeed, the former industrialised areas of the North still have a lower life expectancy: three years lower than the average (ONS, 2019a).

Uneven health performance across the regions has been a distinct feature of the North of England since the national statistics body started to collect

Table 1. Summary statistics of latest life expectancy estimates; UK, constituent countries and regions, 2016 to 2018

	Males			Females		
	Life Expectancy in 2016 to 2018 (years)	Change since 2013 to 2015		Life Expectancy in 2016 to 2018 (years)	Change since 2013 to 2015	
		Months	Weeks		Months	Weeks
UK	79.3	* 1.7	7.4	82.9	* 1.1	4.6
England	79.6	* 2.0	8.8	83.2	* 1.3	5.4
North East	77.9	0.7	3.0	81.7	1.7	7.3
North West	78.3	* 2.3	9.9	81.9	1.1	4.7
Yorkshire and the Humber	78.7	1.3	5.5	82.4	1.0	4.3
East Midlands	79.4	1.8	7.9	82.9	-0.5	-2.2
West Midlands	78.9	1.5	6.5	82.7	-0.1	-0.4
East	80.3	-0.1	-0.6	83.7	0.2	1.0
London	80.7	* 5.9	25.6	84.5	* 5.6	24.5
South East	80.7	* 2.3	9.9	84.1	* 1.6	7.1
South West	80.2	1.3	5.5	83.8	-0.2	-1.0
Wales	78.3	-1.4	-6.0	82.3	0.4	1.7
Scotland	77.1	-0.7	-3.0	81.1	-0.6	-2.7
Northern Ireland	78.7	* 4.3	18.9	82.4	1.0	4.2

Source: ONS, 2019a

data on local area life expectancy in the 1840s and little has changed since then. Southern areas still outperform northern areas in life expectancy. Life expectancy has continued to rise in some regions, but has actually stalled in others. The ONS reported small increases in male and female life expectancy at birth in the UK between 2013 to 2015 and 2016 to 2018 (0.2% and 0.1% respectively). However even in the regions where there were increases, these were substantially smaller than those reported during the first decade of the 21st century. In fact, only England and Northern Ireland reported any significant improvements in life expectancy at birth between 2013 to 2015 and 2016 to 2018. Remaining consistent with previous observations, life expectancy at birth remained highest in the four most southerly regions of England in 2016 to 2018 for both males and females (ONS, 2019a).

In addition, ONS data reported that England had the highest life expectancy at birth and Scotland the lowest in the UK. The gap was not as significant as the overall inter-regional gap within countries, but it stood at 1.9 years for males between England and Scotland and 1.7 years for women in 2018 (ONS, 2019b).

Life expectancy figures and premature deaths are not the only measures to be taken into account when comparing health outcomes in regions. Another very important factor to take into consideration is the actual health of the population and, in particular, the number of years that the population can expect to live in good health. On this account the North also fares badly compared to the Southern regions, with fewer years spent living in good health (ONS, 2019b). The gap between local areas for healthy life expectancy has been reported to be large and growing with the gap amounting to 18.6 years between the highest and lowest performing region in the UK. The areas with the lowest healthy life expectancy are in localities of South Wales, Eastern Scotland, Northern Ireland and the North of England. Blackpool in the North West of England is reported as having the lowest healthy life expectancy at birth for men in the UK. On average, men in this locality can only expect to live 53.3 years in good health. Richmond-upon-Thames has the highest healthy life expectancy, that of 71.9 years (ONS, 2019b). Areas with poor health have remained so over time with similar levels of inequalities in 2009 (Health Foundation, 2020). There are also significant health inequalities in Wales: Blaenau Gwent has the lowest healthy life expectancy and Monmouthshire the highest, with a 10.9 year gap. In Scotland, the gap is even greater between the lowest healthy life expectancy reported in Glasgow City and the highest in East Dunbartonshire, amounting to a 13.6 year gap. Northern Ireland also reports a high gap of 11 years between the lowest healthy life expectancy in Belfast and the highest in Lisburn and Castlereagh (ONS, 2019b).

Other measures include cancer incidence and mortality rates, infant mortality, drug use, alcohol consumption, smokers, chronic diseases and obesity and, in all these areas, regions of the North tend to perform poorly compared to those of the South. In order to be able to tackle such health inequalities, it is important to consider the causes of such disparities between regions and sub-regions.

Determinants of Health Inequalities

A vast literature has been written on the determinants of health inequalities in the hope that this knowledge may further policies to reduce disparities in regions and localities. At an international level, the World Health Organisation (WHO) looks at worldwide social determinants of health and health equity.

Socio-Economic Status and Ill Health

One of the key determinants of inequalities identified by researchers in the field over several decades is the link between low income and ill health. In 2012, the WHO Assembly resolution endorsed the Rio Political Declaration on Social Determinants of Health. It highlighted the need to take into account and act on social determinants of health in all sectors and not just healthcare institutions. In Britain, Richard Wilkinson (1986, 1991, 1994, 1996, 1999, 2003, 2005, 2008) has devoted his career to exploring the question of inequalities, poverty and the link between poverty and ill health. He established a clear link between income inequality and life expectancy. His research shows how serious health inequalities are due to low social status. A number of other studies have confirmed this body of research (Black, 1982; Law and Morris, 1998; Singh and Siahpush, 2006; Wilkinson & Pickett, 2008; Bartley & Blane, 2008; Department of Health, 2009; Dorling, 2013; Inquiry Panel 2014). Michael Marmot's work (Marmot, 2010) also shows that those with low status jobs are more at risk from ill health. Growing inequality in income has thus produced growing inequalities in health. The least deprived can expect to lead 80% of their lives in good health compared to 70% for the most deprived (ONS, 2016a).

But how can inequalities in income lead to poor health? How does low income and low socio-economic status lead to poorer health outcomes? Bartley and Blane established four major models to explain these trends (Bartley & Blane, 2008):

- The Behavioural model: Social class will determine whether an individual's way of life is health damaging or health promoting according to dietary choices, consumption of drugs, alcohol and tobacco, active leisure time pursuits, and use of immunisation, contraception and antenatal services. Nevertheless, long-term studies (n.f. Whitehall study) have found that these differences can only account for one-third of social class differences in mortality. A study by Law and Morris (1998) looking at the factors responsible for differences in mortality between the north and south concluded that while deprivation was the overriding factor, excess mortality was also linked to heavy smoking (in 85% of cases) and heavy alcohol consumption (but only in 6% of cases). The overall consensus among researchers on alcohol consumption is that poorer communities tend to suffer from greater degrees of harm from alcohol consumption, even though the overall consumption level was not found to be higher than in more affluent communities (Erskine, Maheswaran, Pearson, & Gleeson, 2010; Grittner, Kuntsche, Graham, & Bloomfield, 2012; Johnston, Ludbrook, & Jaffray, 2012; Smith, 2013). Finally, Buck found that unskilled males are five times more likely to lead unhealthy life-styles than professional males (Buck, 2014).

- The Materialist model: Poverty leads to greater health hazards. Those suffering from multiple deprivation will most likely be living in polluted environments: inner cities, with greater air pollution and damp housing. The Black Report argued that this was the most important reason for social class differences in health (Black, 1982). According to a recent report, those who live in houses which are cold or damp suffer from poor mental and physical health. The NHS spends at least £2.5 billion a year treating people with illnesses related to cold, damp and dangerous houses. Moreover, people in debt are found to be three more times likely to have mental health problems than those holding no debt (Inquiry Panel, 2014).
- The Psycho-social model: In the more disadvantaged groups, stress may be caused by social stigma or by imbalance between effort and reward; workers in these groups tend to be in jobs where demands are high and control is low. Such stressful working conditions have been linked to high blood pressure, fibrinogen and a more adverse blood fat profile. Lack of job satisfaction at the lower end of the job market is thus seen to have an influence on health.
- The Life-course model: Health is a reflection of the patterns of social, psycho-social and biological advantages and disadvantages experienced by an individual over time. Disadvantages often accumulate through childhood and adulthood. More than ever before, individuals coming from a poor background are likely to experience occupational disadvantage. Children born to disadvantaged families in the UK are more likely to die in the first year of life, be born small, be passive smokers, have weight problems, have children young and die earlier, be out of work, live in poor housing and suffer from poor health.

As the Marmot review of health inequalities in England concluded:

Disadvantage starts before birth and accumulates throughout life. Action to reduce health inequalities must start before birth and be followed through the life of the child. Only then can the links between early disadvantage and poor outcomes throughout life be broken. (Marmot, 2010, p.20)

If we relate these findings on the relationship between low income and poor health outcomes back to the regions, we can conclude that the reason why the North suffers more from poor health is essentially because there is a greater concentration of poverty. Indeed, while there are some affluent areas in the North, it is important to note that the majority of the poorest neighbourhoods are located here. Danny Dorling of the University of Sheffield describes these essential differences in poverty levels, stating that in the north, there are "islands of affluence in a sea of poverty", but "in the south, the sea is of affluence" (quoted in The Economist, 2012).

After 2008, these inequalities worsened. The financial crisis and the loss of jobs, welfare reforms and housing reforms resulted in widening inequalities, leading at the same time to an increase in inequalities in health. Cuts to welfare have impacted on the health of the people receiving those benefits. In particular, those on incapacity benefit, who generally already suffer from ill health, have seen their income decline. Individuals on these benefits lost an average £3,500 with the switch from Disability Living Allowance to Personal Independence Payments which was phased in from 2013 onwards (Inquiry Panel, 2014). Given that the number of people on benefits is higher in the Northern regions, this is likely to produce widening health inequalities for the future. In addition, cuts to housing benefit have a similar effect on health. Children have also been affected by the austerity measures, which raises fears that the health deterioration over a lifetime described above may escalate. Indeed, austerity measures have hit children the hardest due to changes to the welfare and benefits system, such as the abolition of the education maintenance allowance, health in pregnancy grants and child trust funds. Child benefits were frozen in the new round of welfare cuts of 2013 and a number of child centres have been closed in local authorities, but to be fair, London has fared worst, suffering from one fifth of the closures. Child poverty has continued to rise. Almost a third of children in the UK live in poverty owing to rising prices, cuts to benefits and dwindling availability of emergency funds for impoverished families (The Children's Society, 2019).

Industrialisation and Deindustrialisation

A body of research has thus established a clear link between ill health and deprivation. Nevertheless, the link is not necessarily so straightforward. Law and Morris (1998) set out to investigate why higher mortality rates were reported in poorer areas and, especially, more northern areas of England and Wales. They built on previous research which had demonstrated that areas with similar levels of deprivation and socio-economic characteristics report similar health outcomes. Their findings revealed that rural areas and prosperous local authorities had the lowest deprivation and highest life expectancies, urban fringe and coastal and service authorities reported average performance, and mining, manufacturing and industrial (or former mining and manufacturing) areas had the lowest life expectancies and highest levels of deprivation. London was an exception with high and low life expectancies regardless of deprivation. The most deprived areas with the lowest life expectancy could be found in the North, North East and also London. They concluded that there was indeed a link between deprivation and ill health. The populations living in the poorest and most deprived areas did report poorer health. However, it was particularly manual workers or former manual workers in manufacturing and mining sectors that tended to be predisposed towards ill health. The North West for example was reported to have by far the lowest life expectancy. While this region has some very deprived neighbourhoods, it is not the most deprived region of the UK. In fact, mining, manufacturing and industrial local authorities report lower life expectancies than predicted by their levels of deprivation.

The numerous publications on determinants of health inequalities should have effectively encouraged successive governments in the UK to react and formulate policies to try to mitigate inequalities in health performance.

Government Policy to Mitigate Local Health Inequalities

The very first government publication on health inequalities was the Black Report, commissioned by the Labour government but published just after the election of the Conservative government under Margaret Thatcher in 1980 (Black, 1982). It showed that health inequalities were widening and it pointed to the link between social deprivation and poor health outcomes. However, no action was taken by the Conservative government on these issues. It was only in 1998 with the publication of the Acheson report that health inequalities were given real attention (Acheson, 1998).

Sir Donald Acheson, a former Chief Medical Officer, was commissioned by the New Labour government in 1997 to chair an inquiry on health inequalities in England since the mid-1970s and to identify areas where policy development was necessary and likely to reduce inequalities. The independent inquiry was set up after a number of reports showed that, despite increases in living standards and a reduction in mortality in England, the health gap had widened across different socio-economic groups. The report made 39 recommendations to improve health, but also to develop policies to tackle the socio-economic determinants of health. The New Labour government then developed a strategy taking into consideration these recommendations.

New Labour developed a health inequality strategy which was heralded as one of the first, most highly developed and well-funded strategies among European countries to deal with health inequalities. It was a far-reaching strategy going beyond the realm of health. The policies in this framework included raising living standards, improving school nutrition and housing insulation, higher benefits and pensions, more spending on education and urban regeneration as well as increased spending on healthcare. Targets were set to reduce infant mortality and life expectancy inequalities by 10% by 2010 (Department of Health, 2009). A total of £20 billion was allocated to reducing health inequalities and an area approach was taken to deal with these challenges. A spearhead group was established, which contained 70 local authority areas reporting the worst health and deprivation in the country. Higher budgets and targets were established to reduce health inequalities. These areas were primarily in the North, the West Midlands and parts of London (Department of Health, 2009).

While New Labour might be commended for giving attention to health inequalities for the first time in the history of England, and specifically targeting northern areas suffering from deprivation and ill health, there were a number of weaknesses in the policy approach. While there were targets for reducing inequalities in life expectancy and infant mortality, no policies directly addressed income inequality, working conditions or excessive alcohol consumption. Many of the policies were aimed at improving access to treatment but not inequalities or inequities in access. A number of the policies were interlinked with other areas indirectly influencing health such as education, but for which it was impossible to establish the impact on health when considering policy effectiveness. Targets were chosen without first taking into consideration the policies which would be required to achieve such targets. Unfortunately, they were not met. All areas, including the spearhead groups, did see life expectancy rise and infant mortality decrease. However, differences in inequalities in health were not reduced because the spearhead groups simply improved in line with the general population (Department of Health, 2009). The 2010 Marmot review claimed that this was because the targets were not ambitious enough (Marmot, 2010). In particular, the life expectancy and infant mortality targets failed to capture the social gradient in health or the more complex patterning of health associated with other groups (such as ethnic groups). Moreover, the mortality targets did not reflect health status or other dimensions of wellbeing through the life course. Equally, it may have been the case that the targets were perhaps quite simply too ambitious. Yet it is of course possible that health inequalities might have widened without such policies.

In any case, the strategy came to an end in 2010 under the Conservative/ Liberal Democrat coalition government. Nevertheless, the Marmot review, published in 2010, following the implementation of the biggest austerity cuts by the government since the Second World War, underlined that reducing health inequalities remained an important issue, not only to uphold the public good (what the report refers to as a strong social justice case) but also economically, with health costing over £30 billion a year in lost productivity and welfare costs (Marmot, 2010). Following the Health and Social Care Act 2012, the government allocated a ring-fenced public health budget to local authorities to devote to poverty-related health needs, totalling 3% of local government expenditure. However, at the same time, the core local budget was cut by 30%. This obviously was insufficient to tackle health inequalities. Welfare reform, with cuts to local budgets totalling £5.2 billion, has also led to a large financial loss for local economies (Inquiry Panel, 2014). Moreover, since this prevention remit has been removed from the responsibility of the NHS, it would seem that it is very difficult to uphold previous preventative health campaigns. Yet the NHS does have an important role to play in reducing inequalities in health and especially healthcare provision.

The NHS's Role in Ensuring Equity of Supply

In terms of poverty reduction, the distributive effects of public transfers for health are massive. Without the provision of free healthcare, the UK would be second only to Spain on income inequality. By making health payments in kind, income inequalities are reduced by 13%, which means that the UK ranks above the Republic of Ireland and Italy, where rationing of health services has been much more significant (Buck & Jabbal, 2013). The NHS also plays a role as a major regional employer and is, in fact, the biggest employer in Europe (see Table 2).

Table 2. The Biggest Employers in the World (in terms of numbers of employees)

Employer's Name	Number of Employees
US Department of Defense	3.2m
People's Liberation Army, China	2.3m
Walmart	2.1m
McDonald's	1.9m
National Health Service, UK	**1.7m**
China National Petroleum Corporation	1.6m
State Grid Corporation of China	1.5m
Indian Railways	1.4m
Indian Armed Forces	1.3m
Hon Hai Precision Factory (Foxconn)	1.2m

Source: World Economic Forum, Forbes, 2015

The NHS counters poverty by employing not only medical and related staff but also one million non-medical staff. NHS trusts are also committed to providing good quality and decently paid work. This is why an increasing number of NHS trusts are signing up to pay the living wage: Wiltshire Ambulance Trust, Barts Health NHS Trust, the Royal College of Midwives, Derbyshire Community Health Services, and the Chartered Society of Physiotherapy. There are also many schemes in the NHS to help the disadvantaged and long-term unemployed to get back to work. Guy's and St Thomas' Foundation Trust for example runs a range of programmes, including a 'get into work with the NHS' scheme with the Princes Trust, which targets NEETs (Not in employment, education or training) aged 16-to-24 (Buck & Jabbel, 2013).

However, the impact on overall inequality reduction of healthcare is not as significant as might be hoped. Researchers at the Centre for Health Economics, University of York, carried out a longitudinal study for the period 2004/5 to 2011/12 and measured slope indices of inequality in four indicators: patients per family doctor, primary care quality, preventable emergency, hospital admissions and mortality from conditions considered amenable to healthcare. They noted larger absolute improvements on all indicators in more deprived neighbourhoods. By 2011/2012, inequalities in primary care supply and quality were almost eliminated, but socio-economic inequality was still associated with 158,396 preventable hospitalisations and 37,983 deaths amenable to healthcare. The authors concluded that while the NHS did substantially reduce socio-economic inequalities in primary care access and quality, it actually only made modest reductions to healthcare outcome inequalities. Nevertheless, other research carried out to assess the impact of New Labour's inequalities framework has shown that between 2001 and 2011, the increase in resources allocated to deprived areas did enable the reduction of absolute health inequalities from causes amenable to healthcare. Between the aforementioned period, the increase in NHS resources to deprived areas was reported to account for a reduction in the gap between deprived and affluent areas in male mortality amenable to healthcare of 35 deaths per 100,000 population (95% confidence interval 27 to 42) and female mortality of 16 deaths per 100,000. This was reported to explain 85% of the total reduction of absolute inequality in mortality amenable to healthcare during this time (Barr, 2014). Unfortunately, as we mentioned previously, such initiatives and investment have been axed.

Inequities in healthcare remain because there is a so-called "inverse-care law", with good medical care in areas where there is less need. More affluent groups tend to use specialist hospital services more than lower income groups. Access is thus often restricted for lower socio-economic groups. Early studies on the validity of the so-called 'inverse care law' suggested a very wide pattern of inequity in utilisation of services. The term was first used by Tudor Hart, a GP in Wales (Tudor Hart, 1971). Le Grand supported Tudor-Hart's analysis after combining data on the utilisation of services and finding that higher social groups tended to benefit more from healthcare than lower social groups (Le Grand, 1978). However, more recent research suggests that lower income groups tend to consult GP services as often, if not more, than richer groups (Goddard & Smith, 2001). The 'inverse care law' thus tends to be limited to specialist care or inpatient treatment, where richer socio-economic groups are more likely to use these services. Some research has also suggested that there is also an 'inverse care law' in preventative medicine and access to care for chronic diseases. Goddard and Smith (2001) give several reasons for reduced access to healthcare for lower socio-economic groups: 1) Availability: it would seem that some healthcare services are restricted among population groups and clinicians may offer different treatment depending on the population groups, even if needs are identical; 2) the quality of services may vary according to the socio-economic group; 3) costs may differ, although this is not usually the case with the NHS for most services; and 4) healthcare organisations may not enable all population groups to have access to available services. The problem may also lie with the GP mandatory referral procedure. It may be that richer socio-economic groups tend to be more articulate and able to express and request needs to their GP more easily than lower socio-economic groups for more rapid referral to specialists.

Since the implementation of austerity measures in 2010, the rise in health expenditure has slowed down and resources allocated to health inequalities policy have been abolished in many regions, hitting the poorest areas hardest.

The transfer of a certain number of public health responsibilities to local government in England has reduced the role of the NHS in tackling health inequalities, while as we mentioned earlier local governments find their capacities to deal with the wider determinants of health restricted because of budget constraints. Transferring responsibilities from PCTs to CCGs in England has also meant that health inequalities are not necessary focused on in the same way. Under this new framework, quality of health services seems to be of major importance. Integrating health and social care services has also been their priority above targeting certain populations. This can indeed lead to an uneven supply of healthcare across the country. The next section will thus consider regional and inter-regional differences in performance across the UK.

PERFORMANCE OF THE NHS IN THE FOUR NATIONS

To assess the weight and effectiveness of healthcare services in an economy a certain number of indicators are necessary. The traditional indicators that measure value in an economy are added value (or GDP), employment and productivity. However, these traditional indicators only partially reflect the performance of services and are clearly insufficient to measure the performance of health services in an economy.

In line with many other services, it is important to note that healthcare services are more pluri-dimensional than goods sold on the market. Improvement in health tends to be more qualitative than quantitative and it is substantially more difficult to measure qualitative changes than quantitative ones. If qualitative changes are underestimated (which is often the case), the effectiveness of the health system is underestimated. Health services have continued to grow at one of the fastest rates among all goods and services. They have become significant both in terms of value added and employment. They are in fact one of the few areas of activity that have not known a slowdown since the crisis. However, in essence, public services cannot really be measured in terms of their value added. It is very difficult to measure performance in terms of inputs and outputs, so at least value added and productivity have very little meaning in public health services. How can we measure, for example, the performance of a doctor? Should it be in terms of the patients he consults, the treatment or the results? The results will not just depend on the capabilities of the doctor to treat the patient adequately but also the overall health status of the patient and his or her responsiveness to treatment and the effective aftercare the patient receives (Gadrey, 1996; Dalingwater, 2015). Notwithstanding these difficulties in measuring the performance of public health services, a number of statistical measures have been established to compare and contrast performance of health services.

From an international perspective, while the World Health Organisation (WHO) has been rather reluctant in recent times to perform a full-scale comparative analysis of countries' performances in health, they have, nevertheless, underlined the importance of producing measures in order to improve health systems and make governments more accountable for providing sound public health systems. The WHO report *Performance Measurement for Health System Improvement* (Smith, Mossialos & Papanicolas, 2008) reiterates that major improvements are still needed in terms of data collection, analytical methodologies, policy development and implementation of health system performance measurement. It underlines that while satisfactory indicators have been developed for measuring acute hospital care, other areas such as primary care, population health, mental health, financial protection and health system responsiveness research still need to be developed further. The report also assesses the use of targets and their effectiveness as an incentive mechanism to improve health delivery.

Efforts to measure performance of health services originated at least 250 years ago, although a more formalised process introduced by Florence Nightingale and Ernest Codman dates back around 100 years. Nevertheless, the process of assessment has met with professional and political resistance ever since such processes have been introduced. However, health system and health service measurements have developed over the last few decades because of increasing pressures to contain costs, greater demand from patients to have information about treatment and professional audit and accountability. Information technology has also facilitated the collection, processing and dissemination of medical statistics and information. However, many of the performance indicators and health statistics remain at the experimental stage and continuing complexities may thwart adequate production of health service measurements.

In terms of measuring the health of a population and indeed whether health services are adequate in a given country, traditional measures tend to include calculating mortality rates, life expectancy and years of life lost. However, these do not necessarily tell us how health systems are performing. It is difficult, as mentioned earlier, to gauge the extent to which such health outcomes depend on the public health services provided in a country. Another more direct way of measuring effectiveness of health services has been to examine post-treatment mortality, although this depends on the patient's health status before the operation. Clinical outcome measures tend to be the favoured measures to assess the effectiveness of public health service delivery. Another measure is that of analysing the effectiveness of process whether it be monitoring for diseases. A final measure of effectiveness is responsiveness, which is one area that still needs to be developed further for reliability. This essentially refers to evaluating levels of satisfaction with public health services and the general system amongst patients, carers and the general public. It may include waiting time, convenience, easy access, quality of treatment, personal preferences and values. However, responsiveness is often independent of real health outcomes. Finally, productivity measures are often applied to health services, but remain highly challenged because of the difficulties to assess inputs and outputs in healthcare services.

However, in light of recent fiscal constraints and the need to reduce the burden on taxpayers, value for money has become an increasingly important factor and there is pressure to evaluate productivity or at least efficiency of public healthcare services. Patients often vary in terms of the severity of the disease, socio-economic status and life-style behaviour and compliance with treatment recommendations, which makes it very difficult to gauge direct performance comparisons or to detect improvements. The complexity of health systems makes it very hard to summarise performance. Moreover, the wealth of indicators in health services relating to efficiency, equity, quality, responsiveness and access can also make it difficult to summarise health performance because of conflicting accounts. Increasingly, the trend has been to combine performance indicators for comparisons at the country level. However, this also means that a selection of indicators is made with different weights according to significance. Some of the combined indicators will include aspects which are easier to measure than others. However, performance indicators tend to be collected according to targets, which are in essence selective and may result in neglecting untargeted areas. Performance indicators are also used to provide incentives to service providers to improve performance. However, if measurement is not correctly controlled or incentives misdirected, it can make the data unreliable. In short, alongside the technical difficulties of measuring performance of public health services, political considerations must also be taken into consideration.

More specifically, measures of healthcare services tend to be centred on:

- Patient satisfaction and experience and patient reported outcome measures. Patient surveys aim to capture satisfaction and experience.

- Quality of healthcare measured in terms of process as well as outcomes. External organisations tend to be used to assess quality of healthcare.
- Quantity or productivity of healthcare organisations are assessed in terms of patients, bed occupancy and waiting times.
- Financial performance is now considered a key aspect of healthcare performance.

A key focus in the measurement of health systems is quality. However, the definition of quality is a rather nebulous term and interpreted differently depending on the country and/or organisation. In 2001, the US Institute of Medicines (IOM) defined quality healthcare as "safe, effective, patient-centred, timely, efficient and equitable healthcare" (Institute of Medicine, 2001). This definition was also used by the annual US National Healthcare Quality Report and the National Healthcare Disparities Report, to develop similar dimensions of quality. The Organisation for Economic Co-operation and Development (OECD) on the other hand, which produces comparative healthcare indicators in OECD countries, defines quality healthcare as healthcare which ensures effectiveness, safety and is patient-centred (OECD, 2020).

Despite these difficulties in finding effective measures for healthcare, publishing performance indicators is a way of driving improvements provided that they are adequately applied. The first question is to assess how many indicators should be used. Too few indicators could lead to oversimplifying or missing out some important aspects of care. Too many indicators could make it confusing and difficult to read the results. It is also important to consider what kinds of indicators are necessary. Donabedian (1988) suggests three basic types of indicator for measuring the quality of healthcare: structure, process and outcomes. Structure relates to attributes such as nurse/patient ratio, process describes the care administered and outcomes the results after the care has been administered. However, it is important to monitor the reliability of data.

Given the different methodology in measuring health services, the main question is how well do NHS institutions perform across the four nations of the United Kingdom according to the various measures which have been developed.

Performance in the UK From a Global Perspective

From an international perspective, the Commonwealth Fund has consistently ranked the UK first out of 11 other countries. However, other reports show that the UK compares less favourably with other developed countries. Comparing health performance is very difficult. The WHO has refused to analyse and rank health systems since 2000 because it believes it is too complex a process. When assessing the performance of healthcare systems, it is important to bear in mind that the success of these systems depends on life-style and cultural differences, and this means that outcomes will clearly be affected by such differences. Nevertheless, international surveys, such as those carried out by the OECD, have identified certain weaknesses in acute care in the UK. Along with Chile and Poland, the UK is reported to be lagging behind in terms of survival following different diagnoses of cancer (OECD, 2015). Staff have been reported to be too rushed to improve levels of care that have, in many areas, fallen below countries such as Turkey, Portugal and Poland. In 2015, the OECD reported that almost 75,000 more doctors and nurses are needed to match standards in similar countries (OECD, 2015). Since the 2015 report, little has improved. The United Kingdom still has fewer doctors and nurses serving the population than in many OECD countries (2.8 doctors and 7.8 nurses per 1000 population, compared with respective OECD averages of 3.5 and 8.8) (OECD, 2019).

While access to healthcare in the UK is considered to be comparatively good, the quality of care is reported to be mediocre to poor in a number of key health areas (different types of cancer, high rates of smoking, alcohol consumption) and for tackling obesity (64% of adults are overweight or obese in the UK compared to an average of 56% in the OECD (OECD, 2019). The UK was rated 20th out of 35 countries on heart attacks. Nevertheless, the UK was said to perform well on out-of-pocket spending and unmet care needs. Waiting times for planned interventions such as hip and knee replacement were reported to be low and coverage of vaccinations above the OECD average. The OECD's overall conclusions were that too many lives were lost through low quality care and that the UK was not delivering high-quality acute care. The organisation attributed these results partly to under-investment since 2010. Finally, the OECD noted that although the UK has pioneered measurement of quality of health services, actual performance across the health system in the UK remained variable (OECD, 2016; OECD, 2019).

Finally, the Euro Consumer Health Index ranked Britain 15th in Europe for effective healthcare. In particular, it criticised Britain for poor accessibility and an autocratic top-down management culture (Health Consumer Powerhouse, 2018). Indeed, the involvement of an increasing number of managers after the introduction of New Public Management (NPM) would seem to have reinforced a top-down approach and resulted in increased inefficiencies.

An added difficulty for many modern health systems, despite the scarce information in this area, would appear to be the ability to join up or integrate different types of care. The UK is lagging behind in terms of long-term care with one in five people over 50 having to act as informal carers owing to the lack of high quality care (OECD, 2019). International comparisons show how well the UK's health system is performing on a global basis despite the aforementioned measurement difficulties. However, it masks regional and inter-regional differences, which we will turn to next.

Performance in England

Reports on how the NHS in England is performing have tended to point to a rather poor performance in relation to key indicators: notably waiting times, referrals and patient views on care. NHS England figures show one of the worst performances in 2019 in terms of waiting time targets since targets were set. For example, in 2019, it has been reported that the highest number of people since 2004 waited for more than four hours in Accident and Emergency (A&E) and the highest number of people since 2008 waited for essential non-urgent hospital treatment. Moreover, targets for treatment of cancer patients (within 62 days of GP referral) have not been met and there are lengthy delays even to secure a GP appointment (Thorlby, Gardner, & Turton, 2019). For the Health Foundation, this is a sign of more people needing treatment than the NHS can deliver as a result of under-funding, workforce shortages and growing health demands of the population. Cuts to local authority budgets since 2010 (as much as 30% in some localities) have meant extra pressure on public health budgets (preventative health now being the remit of local authorities).

To some extent, guidance as to how well the NHS is performing can actually come from the patients themselves. Both the British Social Attitudes Survey and NHS England's national GP patient survey include performance questions to which patients are invited to respond. For example, the NHS GP patient survey asks 'Overall, how would you describe your experience of your GP surgery?' The proportion of English respondents who rated their GP experience as 'fairly' or 'very' good remained steady throughout 2015 and 2016 at 85%. Other questions include those on dentistry services and hospital services. Positive responses in these areas remain comparatively high. On the whole, satisfaction with the NHS in 2016 was above all for the quality of care (65%), care being free at the point of use (59%), and the range of healthcare provided (47%). The minority of patients expressing dissatisfaction with the NHS in 2016 complained about waiting times (54%), a lack of staff (48%), and a lack of funding (45%) (Robertson, 2017).

Performance of the NHS in Wales

David Cameron was once reported as saying that the English-Welsh border was the 'line between life and death' (Morris, Carrell & McDonald, 2016). He seemed to be suggesting that Welsh healthcare providers do not perform as well as their English counterparts. Owing to real-term cuts in healthcare after 2010, some key services have not been made available to patients in Wales. Some drugs, such as those for cancer are hard to obtain, certain operations are limited or have longer waiting lists than in England, for example heart or knee operations. In recent years, Wales has performed worse than England in hitting targets for admitting, transferring or discharging patients within four hours of arriving in A&E units. In recent years, England has performed better in key diagnosis areas such as hernia, pneumonia and heart disease. Such performance is mainly gauged through observations of longer waiting lists. Welsh patients for example have to wait three times as long for hip operations on average than in the UK. However, performance for diagnosis for cancer was similar in England and Wales (BBC, 2018). Nevertheless, most recent reports show that Welsh waiting times are at their worst level ever. In A&E, only 72,1% of patients were seen within four hours compared to a target of 95%. A record number of patients were left waiting more than 12 hours in A&E (BBC, 2020). This has led Welsh Health Minister Vaughan Gething to pledge an additional £10 million on top of the £30m provided to tackle the problem. Ambulance services also missed their targets of responding in time to life-threatening cases (NHS England, 2020). In some localities, the situation is even worse. For example, the Royal Gwent Hospital in Newport was only able to hit waiting times targets for 53% of its patients. In addition, more than 852 patients were reported waiting more than 12 hours in December 2019 (BBC, 2020).

Morris et al. (2016) note, however, that it is important to look beyond the measures of waiting times and consider questions of quality and safety. But such issues are harder to measure. Nevertheless, the Welsh Government has placed greater emphasis on prevention, public health and social care rather than emphasis on systems performance and targets. The Nuffield Trust reported that while waiting times are a concern, Wales is better than other nations of the UK at hospital discharge into safe social environments, perhaps because more efforts have been made to protect social care. They also underline that it is almost impossible to draw comparisons, given that one caters for a population of 54 million (England) and the other three million (Edwards, 2015). Nevertheless, the fact that a number of patients go across the border to England to receive treatment is telling. In 2014-15, it was found that over 350, 000 Welsh residents sought hospital care in England. This is a much higher figure than Scottish or Northern Irish residents who sought hospital care in England during the same period (Morris et al., 2016).

Performance in Scotland

The picture in Scotland is rather mixed. As noted in the previous section, there are significant health issues in Scotland, with Scottish people suffering from poor health and lower healthy life expectancies compared to the rest of the UK. Nevertheless, the country outperforms the rest of the UK in some areas such as A&E waiting lists. While it has not managed to meet the target of 95% either, the number of patients seen within four hours was highest in Scotland standing at 89.9%, compared to 81.5% in England, 75.2% in Wales and 64.7% in Northern Ireland (NHS Digital, 2019). NHS Scotland's share of health in the total budget is higher than the UK average. This has led to better staffing levels, with 76 GPs per 100,000 here compared to a UK average of 60. They also have more qualified nurses and midwives per 1000 population (8.1 per 1000 in Scotland compared to a UK average of 7.9) (Rolewicz & Palmer, 2019). Scotland also has more hospital beds (4.2 per 1,000 population, compared to a UK average of 2.6). However, some essential hospital equipment has not been acquired because of a lack of funding, for example Stereotactic Ablative Radiotherapy, which is for cancer detection. Scotland has also been criticised for its lack of investment in innovative and effective robotic surgery equipment (Morris et al., 2016). Moreover, according to Audit Scotland, current NHS expenditure in Scotland is financially unsustainable and performance has continued to decline in recent years (Audit Scotland, 2018). Indeed, performance in terms of waiting lists has declined even though it is currently performing better than the rest of the UK. Health boards were reported to be struggling to break even and none of them have managed to meet all key targets. For example, only three of Scotland's regional health boards met the target for patients beginning cancer treatment within 62 days of being referred. NHS Lothian was reported to be performing particularly badly and had failed to meet any of the key targets (Audit Scotland, 2018).

Performance in Northern Ireland

Northern Ireland has significant health issues with a large number of long-term ill patients. 29% of residents were reported to have long-term illnesses here, rising to 39% in some of the most deprived areas of Northern Ireland, which is 25% more than those reported in England and Scotland (Information Analysis Directorate, 2016; Morris et al., 2016). Mental health services are reported to be inadequate to meet the number of people suffering from mental illnesses which often date back to the Troubles. Northern Ireland has the highest levels of post-traumatic stress disorder (PTSD) in the UK. The cost of caring for those with poor mental health outcomes amounts to approximately £47 million a year (Morris et al., 2016). Northern Ireland scores less well than the other nations in terms of waiting times in A&E and performance has been declining in recent years. Emergency Department (ED) attendance increased by 15.1% between 2014/15 and 2018/9 and at the same time performance against the four-hour waiting times target declined quite significantly from 77.5% to 69.9%. Moreover, the number of patients waiting longer than 12 hours increased from 3,170 to 25,326. The increase was very significant in Ulster (Department of Health Northern Ireland, 2019).

Besides differences in performance in the devolved regions of the UK, there are also significant inter-regional differences in performance among and within localities.

Inter-regional Disparities in NHS Healthcare Delivery

While it is very difficult to assess performance or inequity of supply in acute, primary or secondary care, NHS England now publishes data on how hospital trusts are performing. Yet it is extremely difficult to manipulate this data and produce sound comparisons between regions and localities. Professor Sir Brian Jarman of Imperial College, using the data produced by the NHS, did in fact devise a method to measure how well hospitals were performing and thus measure inequity in supply. He calculated the Hospital Standardised Mortality Ratio (HSMR), which records the number of patients who die following different procedures in hospitals. His hypothesis was that you can rate hospitals according to the number of post-operative mortalities. Results were published in the media until 2011, but when it came to light that there were failings in care even in some of the top-rated hospitals such methods were given less credit. Hospitals vary in terms of the population they serve: age, poverty levels, geography, lifestyle, etc. and it is therefore very difficult to measure outcomes accurately. Comparing hospital trusts according to their ability to meet targets is perhaps a more effective way of avoiding inadequate comparisons. The BBC has set up a hospital tracker on trusts' abilities to reach targets for cancer, A&E and operations using NHS England data. According to such tracking, two Northern regions score better on the whole. The North East was actually rated as the best performer with the localities in this region: South Tyneside, Gateshead and North Tees/ Hartlepool, ranked second, third and fourth (see Figure 4).

Figure 4. How English Regions Compare on Targets

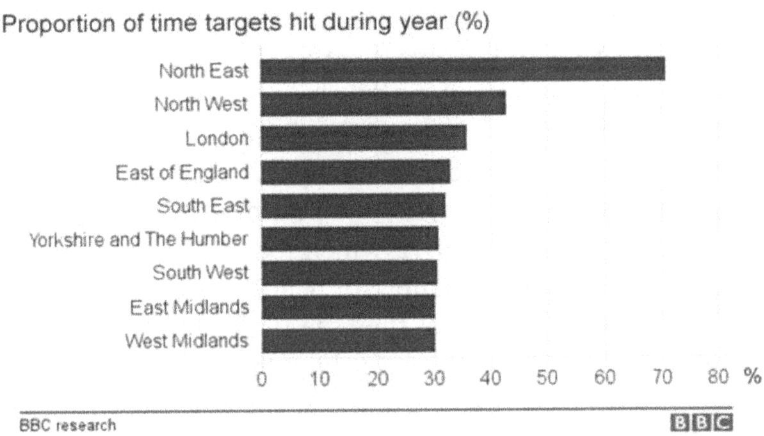

However, this does not tell us about the quality of care received; it just gives information about the hospital trusts' ability to meet targets.

In terms of primary care and the link between acute and primary care, researchers at the University of York noted disparities across the country. The indicators that they used to analyse performance of CCGs focused on emergency hospitalisation for patients with long-term conditions such as dementia, diabetes, respiratory and cardiovascular diseases, which previous research has shown can be reduced by more effective primary and outpatient care. The indicators were part of the NHS England's Clinical Commissioning Group Improvement and Assessment Framework. The results showed that some CCGs are clearly better at tackling health inequalities than others. Some of the most deprived areas of the country performed less well. For example, researchers reported that the Liverpool CCG appears on the worst list as does

Islington. On the other hand, both Portsmouth and Stoke-on-Trent CCGs are seen as the best performers. The latter also belong to the most deprived neighbourhoods in the country. South Cheshire, a wealthy area, performs badly, while East Surrey performs well (Centre for Health Economics, 2016). So, deprived areas are not necessarily the worst performers. Nevertheless, eight of the ten worst performing CCGs in this survey were located in the deprived areas of the North. The best performing CCGs were still largely prosperous areas of the South such as City and Hackney in London, followed by Fareham and Gosport, East Surrey, Crawley and the Isle of Wight (Centre for Health Economics, 2016). Inter-regional differences in healthcare provision were found to be even stronger than regional divides. NHS CCG figures showed for example that patients with dementia, diabetes and learning disabilities received variable care depending on the locality in which they lived. More than half (57%) of CCGs in England were found to be not performing well enough on dementia, with 71% classed as 'needs improvement' for diabetes care and 92% for people with learning disabilities. A total of 149 out of 209 CCGs were reported as needing to improve care for diabetes patients (Centre for Health Economics, 2016). As Matthews (2017) underlines, the Health and Social Care Act of 2012 which led to the setting up of CCGs gave a significant degree of discretion for health services to arrange for the provision of services or facilities as they see fit. This has meant that setting up consistent standards of care across the board is difficult and thus services and resources vary from one CCG to another. CCG service providers can set eligibility and selection criteria for patients for a number of its services and decide to turn away patients.

A study carried out in 2020 also confirmed that deprived areas tend to receive lower quality health services than more affluent areas. The study carried out by Quality Watch found that people living in some of the most deprived areas of England received the worst quality NHS care and also had poorer health outcomes. The joint analysis carried out by Nuffield Trust and the Health Foundation used 23 measures of healthcare quality to assess the link between quality and deprivation. For every single indicator, the level of care received by people with the worst deprivation levels was lower and the gap had increased. Residents of these areas reported spending longer than more affluent areas in A&E and having more difficulties making an appointment to see their local GP (Quality Watch, 2020). In 2014/15 there was no perceivable difference in the percentage of people missing the four hour A&E target between the most deprived areas and the most affluent areas. However, in 2017/18, of the people from the most deprived areas of England who attended A&E, 14.3% were not seen within the target time, whereas the rate was 12.8% in the least deprived areas. Between 2011/12 and 2017/18, respondents from the most deprived areas reporting a 'very good' or 'fairly good' experience when making an appointment to see a GP fell from 77% to 64%, whereas it fell from 81% to 72% in the least deprived areas. The researchers also found significant inequalities in terms of avoidable deaths, smoking prevalence and emergency admissions to hospital. Nevertheless, some measures did show narrowing of inequalities in areas where there have been improvements in care such as unplanned hospital admissions for asthma, diabetes and child epilepsy and recovery rates following psychological therapy (Quality Watch, 2020).

Despite these clear inequities in supply, policy to allocate resources to CCGs does take deprivation into account. Indeed, since 2002, a deprivation adjustment has been made so that CCGs in poorer areas receive larger budgets for the commissioning of primary, community and hospital services. The map in Figure 5 displays these allocations per head across England and it is clear that CCGs in more deprived areas do receive more funding per head:

Scotland, Wales and Northern Ireland have similar policies for deprived localities. However, the House of Commons report contends that this is below what is required if the full healthcare needs of the local populations are taken into consideration. Moreover, despite efforts to continue to take into account deprivation in resource allocation, CCGs lack capacity and population-based data on socio-economic indicators and morbidity, which undermines their ability to achieve equity of access through commissioning (House of Commons, 2014). As the Due North report (Inquiry Panel, 2014) identifies, it is important that the objective of reducing inequalities is upheld by CCGs. Recent policies have perhaps focused too much on solutions for dealing with the aged population at the expense of reducing inequalities. Indeed, the objectives of local health administrators changed after the enactment of the Health and Social Care Act of 2012 in England. Whereas PCTs were specifically engaged in leading local partnerships in order to investigate and address poor health determinants, thus far CCGs have not undertaken this work, or at least not to the same extent as PCTs did. CCGs tend to focus more on developing quality health services and trying to reduce demand for health services (House of Commons, 2014).

However, management of funds across regions is not the only problem, there is also an issue of supply in the regions and sub-regions. Evidence suggests that primary care intervention is crucial in reducing inequalities in life expectancy. The Department of Health estimates that effective primary care

Figure 5. CCG Funding per region in £ per head
Source: House of Commons (2014)

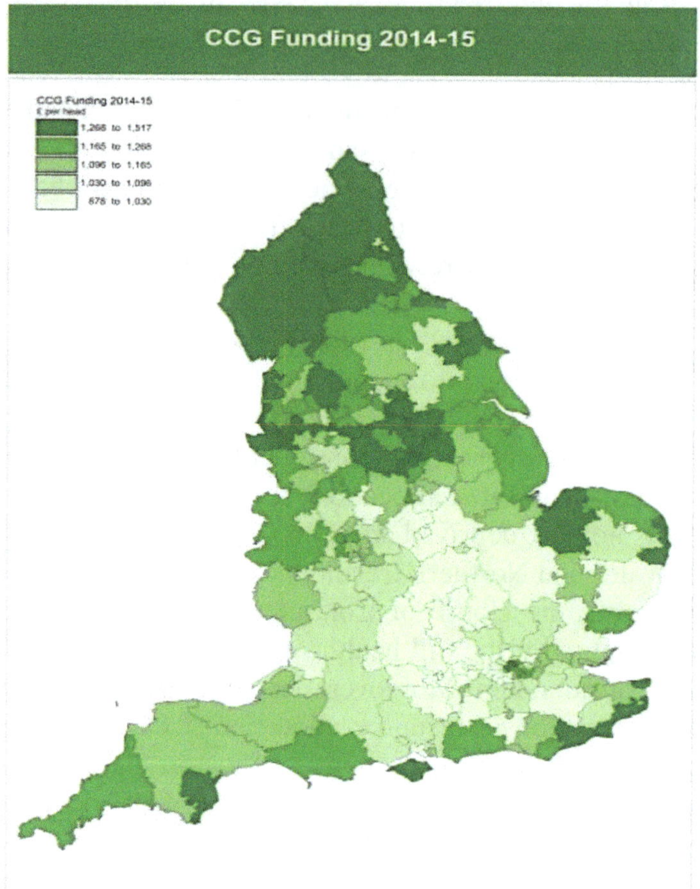

interventions can reduce inequalities by at least 10%. However, the essential problem is that deprived areas suffer even more than other localities from staff shortages. There are fewer than average GPs per head in deprived areas: 56 GPs per 100,000 weighted population, compared to 64 in the wealthiest areas (Buck, 2014). This means that prevention is reduced in the deprived areas.

Faced with the current Covid-19 pandemic, it is clear that the governance framework for the regions and localities will be tried and tested, and could further reinforce some of these underlying local weaknesses.

The NHS' Response to the Covid-19 Pandemic

Despite being in the midst of the Covid-19 outbreak and perhaps lacking hindsight at the time of writing, it would seem appropriate to finish this chapter with a short study of how a global pandemic can have an impact on our national and regional health systems. One of the most salient examples is the current Covid-19 pandemic. Covid-19 refers to a new strain of a large family of viruses (Coronaviruses) which seems to have transferred from animals to humans. There is currently no cure or vaccine to treat or prevent the spread of the virus.

While roughly 80% recover with only mild symptoms, the elderly and those with underlying health risks are most at risk from developing more severe symptoms, which has led to a significant number of deaths worldwide (over 80,000 at the time of writing) with the epicentre currently in Europe and the US (WHO, 2020a).

It was not until 31 December 2019 that the WHO was informed of cases of pneumonia in Wuhan City, China (WHO, 2020a). The WHO did not initially recommend restrictions on travel or trade. Most public health experts, including those working at the WHO, argue that banning travel and trade may be counterproductive and actually hinder information sharing, make it harder to track cases and fuel shortages of drugs and medical supplies in areas hardest hit by the pandemic. The WHO thus set forth guidance on how to prevent and control the spread of the novel virus (WHO, 2020a). The WHO had already adopted a set of International Health Regulations following the SARS epidemic in 2005 in order to establish a legal framework to govern how countries should prepare and respond to outbreaks. At that time, countries were committed to not imposing 'more restrictive' measures than WHO recommendations without providing scientific justification (WHO, 2020a). As the pandemic started to take hold, the WHO stepped up its recommendations which included the need to test more widely and contain the virus by imposing quarantines, stopping movement of people, isolating the sick and tracking down those who might be infected.

As of 6 May 2020, 201,000 confirmed positive cases of Covid-19 have been counted in the UK (including Prime Minister Boris Johnson and some key government ministers) and just over 30,000 have died. While the British government has been criticised for being slow to respond to the Covid-19 outbreak or at least to impose restrictive measures, the government has since stepped up action, in line with WHO recommendations, closing public houses, restaurants, schools and all businesses which are not considered key to the functioning of the country. However, the pandemic is still taking its toll on the NHS and its services are currently overwhelmed with patients suffering from severe cases of the disease.

The WHO made a number of recommendations to ensure that health systems responded adequately to Covid-19 and many of these recommendations required increasing staffing levels:

Table 3. Summary of 16 health system recommendations to respond to COVID-19

1. Expand capacity for communication and proactively manage media relations.	2. Bolster capacity of essential public health services to enable emergency response.	3. Clarify first-point-of-contact strategy for possible COVID-19 cases: phone, online, physical.	4. Protect other potential first-contact health system entry points.
5. Designate hospitals to receive COVID-19 patients and prepare to mobilize surge acute and ICU capacity.	6. Organize and expand services close to home for COVID-19 response.	7. Maintain continuity of essential services while freeing up capacity for COVID-19 response.	8. Train, repurpose and mobilize the health workforce according to priority services.
9. Protect the physical health of frontline health workers.	10. Anticipate and address the mental health needs of the health workforce.	11. Review supply chains and stocks of essential medicines and health technologies.	12. Mobilize financial support and ease logistical and operational barriers.
13. Assess and mitigate potential financial barriers to accessing care.	14. Assess and mitigate potential physical access barriers for vulnerable groups of people.	15. Optimize social protection to mitigate the impact of public health measures on household financial security.	16. Ensure clarity in roles, relationships and coordination mechanisms in health system governance and across government.

Source: WHO (2019b)

Many of these points are the remit of the NHS. Some of the recommendations have indeed been followed. In terms of bolstering capacity, the NHS called retired staff back to support hospitals to respond to emergencies. More than 18,000 doctors, nurses and former NHS staff thus volunteered to return to help combat Covid-19 (NHS UK, 2020). The staff were given full induction and online training to be able to meet current demands to deal with the pandemic. Moreover, a "Your NHS needs you" also led to a further 725,000 people volunteering to help deliver medicines from pharmacies, drive patients to appointments, bring patients home from hospital and make regular phone calls to check on people self-isolating at home (NHS UK, 2020). The NHS also quickly developed the 111 phone and internet service to serve as a first-point of contact. Other specific first contact health system entry points were also established. However, it has been impossible to continue some regular services or designate specific Covid-19 hospitals as recommended by the WHO.

Two new 'nightingale' hospitals have been created to deal specifically with the increase in demand for acute care during the pandemic. One hospital will be based at the NEC in Birmingham with up to 500 beds equipped with the capacity to increase beds up to 2,000 if needed. The other at the Manchester Central Complex will provide up to 500 beds but could expand further to 1,000 beds for coronavirus patients across the North West of England. These hospitals are intended to provide support for patients from across the Midlands and the North West (NHS England, 2020). Moreover, a temporary hospital at East London's ExCel centre has been assembled to bear the brunt of the surge in intensive care patients in the capital. NHS leaders are not planning to transfer patients elsewhere in the country to ensure that Covid-19 can be contained. London is the epicentre of Covid-19 in the UK at the time of writing with 2,000 Covid-19 patients in London hospitals, which represents just under a half of all those in hospital across England. London already has around 800 intensive care beds and a surge capacity of up to 3,000 beds. However, NHS England reported that they estimate needing approximately seven times more, which explains why it was so important to assemble the hospital at the ExCel centre. More field hospitals are likely to be created across England (NHS England, 2020).

The NHS has also reached out to the private health sector for support. It concluded a deal with private hospitals across the country to acquire beds, ventilators and clinicians. The government has also created a consortium including Ford, Siemens and the McLaren and Mercedes Formula 1 teams in order to build new ventilators. (The Economist, 2020)

However, the underlying weaknesses in the NHS: limits to funding, fewer doctors, nurses, hospital beds and equipment (capital investment) in the UK compared with European counterparts suggest that it will prove difficult to respond to all the critical care needs and align responses with the WHO criteria. While protecting the physical and mental health of frontline staff is an essential recommendation, in practice it will prove difficult to follow given the structural weaknesses of the NHS. Hospitals lack sufficient tests to screen frontline staff, which means that 20 to 25% of NHS doctors and nurses have had to self-isolate because of signs of a cough, cold or temperature, which may well be unrelated to the coronavirus. The NHS also lacks sufficient ventilators.

The Covid-19 pandemic has also brought to light essential sub-regional inequalities in healthcare provision. While the full effects of the Coronavirus on the healthcare systems in the UK are yet to be seen at the time of writing, research from Edge Health shows that London is actually better prepared to cope with Covid-19. While London is set to be the hardest hit by the pandemic, all regions are likely to meet with substantial pressures. A significant shortage of acute beds has already been reported. The Edge Health report suggests despite the intended increase in bed capacity, there will still be a shortage. Moreover, the shortage is likely to be most felt in the regions beyond the capital. London has 30% more critical care beds per head of the population, which corresponds to normal demand based on demographics. However, Covid-19 tends to result in higher hospital admissions for the elderly, which means that there is significant pressure in those regions with a higher ratio of older people. These localities also tend to be where there are fewer beds per head of population. (Batchelor, 2020).

Only time will tell how the NHS copes with this global pandemic in light of its structural weaknesses and one of the biggest challenges to its system in living memory.

CONCLUSION

Despite the qualities of a universal health system, which should reduce inequalities in healthcare, it is clear that there are still significant unequal health outcomes and inequity of supply in healthcare across the regions of the UK and within localities. Different governance arrangements may have mitigated the situation to a certain extent, which is notably the case in Scotland, but funding pressures and the limited extent to which health systems alone can improve health outcomes means that these health gains are marginal. Times of crises underline the underlying structural weaknesses and disparities in terms of supply as is evident from the Covid-19 case study. CCGs and their equivalent in the devolved administrations have nevertheless been focusing on the integration of health and social care services, which is one way in which health inequalities between and within regions may be tackled in a more co-ordinated manner. This will be the focus of the next chapter.

REFERENCES

Acheson, D. (1998). *Public health in England: The report of the committee of inquiry into the future development of the public health function*. HMSO.

Appleby, J. (2005). *Independent review of health and social care services in Northern Ireland.* Department of Health, Social Services and Public Safety of Northern Ireland. Retrieved April 5, 2020, from http://www.dhsspsni.gov.uk/appleby-report.pdf

Barr, B., Bambra, C., & Whitehead, M. (2014). The impact of NHS resource allocation policy on health inequalities in England 2001-11: Longitudinal ecological study. *BMJ (Clinical Research Ed.)*, *348*(6), g3231. doi:10.1136/bmj.g3231 PMID:24865459

Bartley, M., & Blane, D. (2008). Inequality and social class. In G. Scambler (Ed.), *Sociology as applied to medicine* (6th ed., pp. 115–132). Saunders Elsevier.

Batchelor, G. (2020, March 19). Revealed: huge regional variation in NHS' ability to meet coronavirus demand. *HSJ*. Retrieved April 10, 2020, from https://www.hsj.co.uk/ quality-and-performance/ revealed-huge-regional-variation- in-nhs-ability-to-meet-coronavirus-demand/ 7027153.article.

BBC News. (2018, January 12). *Reality Check: Is NHS funding worse in Wales?* Retrieved April 3, 2020, from https://www.bbc.com/news/health-42655140

BBC News. (2020, January 23). *A&E: Welsh waiting times hit worst ever level*. Retrieved April 3, 2020, from https://www.bbc.com/news/uk-wales-51209403

Bevan, G., Karanikolos, M., Exley, J., Nollte, E., Connolly, S., & Mays, N. (2014). *The four health systems of the United Kingdom: How do they compare*? Nuffield, Trust/Health Foundation. Retrieved April 5, 2020, from https://www.nuffieldtrust.org.uk/ research/the-four-health-systems- of-the-uk-how-do-they-compare

Black, D. (1982). *Inequalities in health: Black report*. Pelican Series, Penguin Books.

Buck, D. (2014). *How healthy are we? A high-level guide*. King's Fund publication.

Buck, D., & Jabbal, J. (2013). *Tackling poverty: Making more of the NHS in England*. King's Trust.

Centre for Health Economics. (2016, August 16). *NHS adopts Centre for Health Economics Clinical Commissioning Group health inequality indicators*. University of York, Centre for Health Economics, Retrieved May 8, 2018, from: https://www.york.ac.uk/ che/news/2016/ nhs-adopts-che-ccg-indicators/

Dalingwater, L. (2015). *Les services britanniques au 21e siècle: une étude interdisciplinaire*. Presses Universitaires de Nancy.

Dayan, M., & Edwards, N. (2017). Learning from Scotland's NHS. Research Report. Nuffield Trust.

Department of Health. (1997). The new NHS: Modern, dependable. CM 3807. HMSO.

Department of Health. (2000, July). *The NHS plan: A plan for investment, a plan for reform*. Cm 4818-I. HMSO.

Department of Health. (2001). *Shifting the balance of power within the NHS*. Crown.

Department of Health. (2009). *Tackling health inequalities: Ten years on*. HMSO.

Department of Health. (2010). *Healthy lives, healthy people: Our strategy for public health in England*. HMSO.

Department of Health Northern Ireland. (2019, June 21). *Northern Ireland hospital statistics: Emergency care (2018/19)*. Retrieved April 8, 2020, from https://www.health-ni.gov.uk/ news/northern-ireland-hospital-statistics-emergency-care-201819

Donabedian, A. (1988, September 23-30). The quality of care. How can it be assessed? *Journal of the American Medical Association, 260*(12), 1743–1748. doi:10.1001/jama.1988.03410120089033 PMID:3045356

Dorling, D. (2013). *Unequal health: The scandal of our times*. The Policy Press. doi:10.2307/j.ctt1t891pj

Erskine, S., Maheswaran, R., Pearson, T., & Gleeson, D. (2010). Socio-economic deprivation, urban-rural location and alcohol-related mortality in England and Wales. *BMC Public Health, 10*(99). Advance online publication. doi:10.1186/1471-2458-10-99 PMID:20184763

Gadrey, J. (1996). *L'économie des services*. Éditions La Découverte.

Goddard, M., & Smith, P. (2001, November). Equity of access to healthcare services: Theory and evidence from the UK. *Social Science & Medicine*, *53*(9), 1149–1162. doi:10.1016/S0277-9536(00)00415-9 PMID:11556606

Gorsky, M., Lock, K., & Hogarth, S. (2014, December). Public health and English local government: Historical perspectives on the impact of 'returning home'. *J Public Health*, *36*(4), 546–551. doi:10.1093/pubmed/fdt131 PMID:24472776

Greer, S. L. (2004). *Territorial politics and health policy: UK health policy in comparative perspective*. Manchester University Press.

Grittner, U., Kuntsche, S., Graham, K., & Bloomfield, K. (2012, September). Social inequalities and gender differences in the experience of alcohol-related problems. *Alcohol and Alcoholism (Oxford, Oxfordshire)*, *47*(5), 597–605. doi:10.1093/alcalc/ags040 PMID:22542707

Grosios, K., Gahan, P. B., & Burbidge, J. (2010, December). Overview of healthcare in the UK. *The EPMA Journal*, *1*(4), 529–534. doi:10.100713167-010-0050-1 PMID:23199107

Haggerty, J., & Levesque, J. F. (2013). The strength of primary care systems. *BMJ (Clinical Research Ed.)*, *346*(7941). PMID:23766466

Ham, C. (2009). *Health policy in Britain* (6th ed.). Palgrave Macmillan. doi:10.1007/978-1-137-01397-2

Harrington, B., Smith, K., Hunter, D., Marks, L., Blackman, T., McKee, L., Greene, A., Elliott, E., & Williams, G. (2009, January). Health inequalities in England, Scotland and Wales: Stakeholders' accounts and policy compared. *Public Health*, *123*(1), e24–e28. doi:10.1016/j.puhe.2008.10.010 PMID:19084881

Health Consumer Powerhouse. (2018). *Euro Health Consumer Index 2017*. Health Consumer PowerHouse Ltd.

Health Foundation. (2018, June 16). *Health Foundation response to government announcement of additional NHS funding*. Retrieved January 22, 2019, from https://www.health.org.uk/ news-and-comment/news/ health-foundation-response-to-government- announcement-of-additional-nhs-funding

House of Commons. (2014, January 27). *New CCG funding allocations – mapped*. London: House of Commons Library. Retrieved May 18, 2018, from https://secondreading.uk/ author-john-wood/ new-ccg-funding-allocations-mapped/

Information Analysis Directorate. (2016). *Health inequalities, Annual report 2016*. Department of Health Northern Ireland. Retrieved March 26, 2020, from http://www.nisra.gov.uk

Inquiry Panel on Health Equity for the North of England. (2014). *Due North: The report of the inquiry on health equity for the North*. University of Liverpool and Centre for Local Economic Strategies.

Institute of Medicine. (2001). *Crossing the quality chasm: A new health system for the 21st century*. The National Academy of Sciences.

Johnston, M. C., Ludbrook, A., & Jaffray, A. (2012). Inequalities in the distribution of the costs of alcohol misuse in Scotland: A cost of illness study. *Alcohol and Alcoholism (Oxford, Oxfordshire)*, *47*(6), 725–731. doi:10.1093/alcalc/ags092 PMID:22890793

Law, M. R., & Morris, J. K. (1998). Why is mortality higher in poorer areas and in more northern areas of England and Wales? *Journal of Epidemiology and Community Health*, *52*(6), 344–352. doi:10.1136/jech.52.6.344 PMID:9764254

Marmot, M. (2010). *Fair society, healthy lives Marmot review: Strategic review of health inequalities*. Department for International Development.

Matthews, D. (2017). The battle for the National Health Service. *Monthly Review (New York, N.Y.)*, *68*(10), 25. doi:10.14452/MR-068-10-2017-03_3

Ministry of Health. (1946). *A National Health Service*. HMSO.

Morris, S., Carrell, S., & McDonald, H. (2016, February 9). How healthcare differs across the UK. *The Guardian*. Retrieved June 7, 2018, from https://www.theguardian.com/politics/2016/feb/09/how-healthcare-differs-across-the-uk

National Assembly for Wales. (2015). *The organisation of the NHS in the UK: Comparing structures in the four countries*. National Assembly for Wales.

NHS Digital. (2019, September 12). *Hospital accident & emergency activity 2018-19*. Retrieved April 10, 2020, from https://digital.nhs.uk/data-and-information/publications/statistical/hospital-accident--emergency-activity/2018-19

NHS UK. (2020, March 30). *NHS to open two more new hospitals to fight COVID-19*. Retrieved April 4, 2020, from https://www.fyldecoastccgs.nhs.uk/ 2020/03/nhs-to-open-two- more-new-hospitals-to-fight-covid-19/

NHS Wales. (2010). *Five-year service, workforce and financial strategic framework for NHS Wales*. Welsh Assembly Government. Retrieved April 9, 2020, from www.wales.nhs.uk/documents/executive-summary.pdf

NHS Wales. (2011). *NHS Wales delivery framework for 2011/12*. Retrieved April 9, 2020, from www.wales.nhs.uk/ sitesplus/documents/986/nhs%20wales%20delivery%20framework% 20for%20wales%202011-12.pd

OECD. (2015). *Health at a glance*. OECD.

OECD. (2017). *Health at a glance*. OECD.

OECD. (2019). *Health at a glance*. OECD.

OECD. (2020). *Healthcare quality and outcomes*. Retrieved April 15, 2020, from https://www.oecd.org/health/health-care-quality-and-outcomes.htm

ONS. (2016a, November 29). *Health state life expectancies, UK: 2013 to 2015*. ONS. Retrieved September 8, 2017, from https://www.ons.gov.uk/releases/healthstatelifeexpectanciesuk2013to2015

ONS. (2016b, March 10) *Statistical bulletin: Healthy life expectancy at birth and age 65 by upper tier local authority and area deprivation: England, 2012 to 2014*. ONS. Retrieved September 8, 2017, https://www.ons.gov.uk/ peoplepopulationandcommunity/ healthandsocialcare/healthandlifeexpectancies/ bulletins/healthylifeexpectancyatbirthandage65byuppertierlocal authorityandareadeprivation/england2012to2014

ONS. (2019a, December 11). *Health state life expectancies, UK: 2016 to 2018*. ONS. Retrieved April 10, 2020, from https://www.ons.gov.uk/ peoplepopulationandcommunity/ healthandsocialcare/healthandlifeexpectancies/ bulletins/healthstatelife expectanciesuk/2016to2018

ONS. (2019b, December 2). *Past and projected period and cohort life tables, 2018-based, UK: 1981 to 2068*. ONS. Retrieved April 3, 2020, from https://www.ons.gov.uk/peoplepopulationandcommunity/birthsdeathsandmarriages/lifeexpectancies/ bulletins/pastandprojecteddatafromtheperiodandcohortlifetables/ 1981to2068

Parkin, D. (2017). *Principles of health economics*. Retrieved September 8, 2017, from: https://www.healthknowledge.org.uk/ public-health-textbook/medical-sociology-policy-economics/ 4d-health-economics/principles-he

Pollock, A., & Price, D. (2013). Duty to care: In defence of universal healthcare. Policy Paper. London: Centre for Labour and Social Studies.

Pritchard, C., & Wallace, M. (2011). Comparing the USA, UK and 17 Western countries' efficiency and effectiveness in reducing mortality. *Journal of the Royal Society of Medicine*, *2*(7), 60. PMID:21847442

PWC. (2016). *Redrawing the health and social care architecture*. PWC. Retrieved April 8, 2020, from file:///D:/V10866/Documents/ recentchanges/healthpublication/ 2020versionNHS/ health_architecture_SUMMARY.pdf.

Rannan-Eliya, R., & Somanathan, A. (2006). Equity in health and healthcare systems in Asia. In A. Jones (Ed.), *Elgar companion to health economics* (pp. 205–217). Edward Elgar Publishing. doi:10.4337/9781845428914.00029

Robertson, R. (2017). *Public satisfaction with the NHS and social care in 2016*. King's Fund.

Rolewicz, L., & Palmer, B. (2019). *The NHS workforce in numbers*. Nuffield Trust. Retrieved April 2, 2020, from https://www.nuffieldtrust.org.uk/resource/the-nhs-workforce-in-numbers

Scotland, A. (2018, October). *NHS in Scotland 2018*. Audit General. Retrieved April 6, 2020, from https://www.audit-scotland.gov.uk/ uploads/docs/report/2018/nr_181025_nhs_overview.pdf

Singh, G. K., & Siahpush, M. (2006, August). Widening socio-economic inequalities in US life expectancy 1980-2000. *International Journal of Epidemiology*, *35*(4), 969–979. doi:10.1093/ije/dyl083 PMID:16684899

Smith, K. (2013). *Beyond evidence based policy in public health*. Palgrave. doi:10.1057/9781137026583

Smith, P. C., Mossialos, E., & Papanicolas, I. (2008). *Performance measurement for health system improvement: Experiences, challenges and prospects*. European Regional Office for the WHO.

Steel, D., & Cylus, J. (2012). United Kingdom (Scotland): Health system review. *Health Systems in Transition*, *14*(9), 1–150. PMID:23579054

The Children's Society. (2019). *It's hard to believe that there are four million children living in poverty in the UK today*. Retrieved April 9, 2020, from https://www.childrenssociety.org.uk/ what-we-do/our-work/ ending-child-poverty/ what-is-child-poverty

The Economist. (2012, September 15). The great divide. *The Economist*. Retrieved June 5, 2017, from https://www.economist.com/britain/2012/09/15/ the-great-divide

The Economist. (2020, 4 April). Move fast and try not to break things. *The Economist*, 19-20.

The Health Foundation. (2020, February 26). *Regional differences in health are large and growing*. The Health Foundation. Retrieved April 10, 2020, from https://www.health.org.uk/ news-and-comment/ charts-and-infographics/ male-healthy-life-expectancy-from-birth

Thorlby, R., Gardner, T., & Turton, C. (2019, November 22). *NHS performance and waiting times*. Health Foundation. Retrieved April 9, 2020, from https:// www.health.org.uk/ news-and-comment/ blogs/nhs-performance-and-waiting-times

Tudor Hart, J. (1971). The inverse care law. *Lancet*, *1*(7696), 405–412. doi:10.1016/S0140-6736(71)92410-X PMID:4100731

UK Public General Acts. (n.d.). *Health and Social Care Act 2012*. Retrieved June 21, 2017, from http://www.legislation.gov.uk/ukpga/2012/7/contents/ enacted

Wanless, D. (2004). *Securing good health for the whole population*. HMSO.

Watch, Q. (2020, January 23). *Poorest get worse quality of NHS care in England, new research finds*. Retrieved April 9, 2020, from https://www. nuffieldtrust.org.uk/ news-item/ poorest-get-worse-quality-of- nhs-care-in-england-new-research-finds

WHO. (2017). *Glossary of Terms*. Retrieved July 6, 2017, from https://www.who.int/hia/about/glos/en/index1.html

WHO. (2020a). *Country & Technical Guidance - Coronavirus disease (COVID-19)*. Retrieved April 10, 2020, from https://www.who.int/emergencies/diseases/ novel-coronavirus-2019/ technical-guidance

WHO. (2020b). *Strengthening the health system response to COVID-19. Recommendations for the WHO European Region Policy brief*. Retrieved April 10, 2020, from http://www.euro.who.int/__data/assets/ pdf_file/0003/436350/strengthening-health-system-response-COVID-19.pdf

Wilkinson, R. G. (1986). *Class and health: Research and longitudinal data*. Tavistock Publications.

Wilkinson, R. G. (1994). *Unfair shares: The effects of widening income differences on the welfare of the young*. Barnardos.

Wilkinson, R. G. (1996). *Unhealthy societies: The afflictions of inequality*. Routledge.

Wilkinson, R. G. (2005). *The impact of inequality: How to make sick societies healthier*. Routledge.

Wilkinson, R. G., Kawachi, I., & Kennedy, B. P. (1999). *The society and population health reader* (Vol. 1). New Press Distributed by W.W. Norton.

Wilkinson, R. G., & Michael, M. (2003). *The solid facts*. World Health Organization, Regional Office for Europe.

Wilkinson, R. G., & Pickett, K. E. (2008). *Health and inequality: Major themes in health and social welfare*. Routledge.

Wilkinson, R. G., & Quick, A. (1991). *Income and health*. Socialist Health Association.

World Economic Forum. Forbes. (2015, June 17). *Who is the world's biggest employer? The answer might not be what you expect*. Retrieved June 11, 2017, from https://www.weforum.org/agenda/2015/06/worlds-10-biggest-employers/

ENDNOTES

1 Scotland, Northern Ireland and Wales are considered as both nations and regions.

2 The North refers to three regions of England: The North East, the North West and Yorkshire and the Humber. But in some accounts referring to outcomes (but not policies), this also includes Wales, Scotland and Northern Ireland.

3 Health and social welfare functions were actually the responsibility of English local government from Tudor times when parishes were in charge of carrying out these functions. However, on the creation of the NHS in 1948, very limited public health functions were actually granted to local authorities with the creation of a Medical Officer of Health (MOH) and all other hospitals and clinical services became governed by new centralised NHS bodies (Gorsky, Lock, & Hogarth, 2014).

4 As mentioned in Chapter 1, to consult a GP in England, patients must be enrolled in the GP's practice and form part of the list of patients for that practice. British doctors are then paid a set amount for each patient, regardless of whether the patient seeks care or not.

Chapter 6
Integrated Care:
Towards a New Governance Framework

ABSTRACT

Delivering high quality health and social care is considered to be one of the key governance challenges in the UK. People are living longer, and chronic diseases are more prevalent, which puts ever more pressure on health and social services to deliver. In order to better co-ordinate these services and deal with increased demand and funding pressures, authorities at both national and local levels are moving towards integrated care services. However, the integration of these services is plagued with difficulties. This chapter will explore the complexities of joining-up health and social care. It includes a case study of Continuing Healthcare (CHC), which is a package of care provided by the National Health Service (NHS) and which involves a number of providers across the health and social care sectors. While much of the chapter focuses on health and social care challenges in England, it will finish with analysis of Scotland's progress towards integrated services.

INTRODUCTION

Integrated care is a universal concept, although the focus of integrated care depends on the country's healthcare system and practices. It might sometimes be referred to as seamless care[1], transmural care[2], care management and networking. In general, we can observe two larger streams within the integrated care discourse. First, integrated care may refer more generally

DOI: 10.4018/978-1-7998-3928-6.ch006

to 'managed care' and/or 'public health'. Integration of 'managed care' is concerned with the organisational interfaces within the health system while applying respective rationales and principles on primary healthcare and social care services (Leichsenring, 2004). The World Health Organisation (WHO) defines integrated care as:

A concept bringing together inputs, delivery, management and organisation of services related to diagnosis, treatment, care, rehabilitation and health promotion. Integration is a means to improve the services in relation to access, quality, user satisfaction and efficiency (WHO European Office for Integrated Health Care Services, 2001).

The 'public health approach' is centred around the integration between primary and secondary care, and often on both the vertical and the horizontal level, to provide a more effective social service delivery. The particular focus of this kind of 'public health approach' is the hospital versus community care interface. Integration from the public health perspective thus aims at delivering better care by ensuring integration of various providers (Leichsenring, 2004).

Second, integrated care may refer to integrating social and healthcare and/or the integration of the patient into the process of healthcare provision: i.e. a 'person-centred approach' as illustrated in Chapter 4 or a 'whole system approach'. Paying attention to these various processes is expected to enable health services to be co-ordinated more effectively. The 'person-centred discourse' does have something in common with the public health discourse. However, its aim is to show more extensively the interdependence of social and health services in the long term, by putting the individual at the centre of service delivery:

The integration of health and social services implies that the services are provided to all elderly—independent of where they live—by integrated teams of home-helpers, home nurses etc. (...) The decision of support is made on request from GPs, hospitals, the elderly or relatives (Colmorten, Clausen, & Bengtsson, 2004, p. 6).

This is close to what is called 'demand-driven healthcare', meeting the needs of the patient or client by providing integrated care, and is also specifically mentioned in the Care Act of 2014. However, for real integration to take place, a stable organisation would have to provide all coverage for healthcare needs. It might also mean that social services become more medicalised (Leichsenring, 2004).

DELIVERING INTEGRATED CARE IN THE UK

Delivering high quality health and social care is considered to be one of the key challenges that the British government is currently facing. People are living longer and chronic diseases are more prevalent, which puts ever more pressure on health and social services to deliver. In order to better co-ordinate these services and deal with increased demand and funding pressures, authorities at both national and local levels are moving towards integrated care services. There is a wide literature in both the UK and at international level which supports integrated care services (Gagliardi et al., 2014; Cheetham et al., 2017; Ham, 2018b; Charles, Wenzel, Kershaw, Ham, & Walsh, 2018). In the UK, a central lead was taken to integrate health and social care starting primarily with the government commissioned Dilnot blueprint for reform of social care funding, followed by the *NHS Five Year Forward View* (NHS England, 2014), which has recently been followed by a more intensive study of long-term care needs in the *NHS Long-Term Plan* (NHS England, 2019), in which the ambition is that all localities in England would benefit from Integrated Care Systems (ICSs) by April 2021.

However, joining-up the various health services in both primary and secondary settings, and joining-up these services with social services is an extremely complex procedure. It requires the coming together of local government services and the myriad of health organisations in the public, private and third sectors (given that many health and social services are sub-contracted out beyond the public sphere, in England at least). The main problem is that to date there are no statutory arrangements to make ICSs legally binding in England, which means that joining-up services is in fact a voluntary exercise and enacted according to what each locality believes is best for the service users. Whether it be the joining-up of various services within the health sector or health and social care services, a joined-up approach is challenging.

Acute Care vs. Primary Care

The balance between achieving sound acute and primary care is often seen to be quite problematic. Indeed, accusations are often made that the government is primarily interested in the here and now, dealing with acute care rather than preventative measures in a primary care setting. Indeed, acute care continues to receive more funding. Boldt, Dimson and Kloss (2010) report that acute care in a hospital setting usually accounts for 40 to 50% of total health expenditure. The situation may have improved since the Wanless reports, which criticised the government for its preoccupation with acute care and hospital beds, but striking the balance continues to prove difficult. Regional variations and variations between different services have gained wide media coverage. In an attempt to offer the best possible service, the 1997 Primary Care Act was enacted to offer greater flexibility and choice for the patient to choose the primary care provider. The Act also provided for a number of pilot projects: employment of salaried family doctors, nurse schemes, cooperatives of doctors to provide evening and weekend services, etc. In addition, the creation of NHS Direct, a health advice and information service (which was unfortunately discontinued in 2014) and walk-in centres, providing expert advice by nurses for minor injuries, strengthened the provision of primary care. The extension of choice in primary care was further supported by policy prescriptions (Ham, 2009). At the same time acute services still remain a priority in the NHS, especially with medical advances that have helped advance diagnosis and treatment, but also because of expectations on the part of the general public and fuelled by the media. However, *The NHS Five Year Forward (Forward View)* (NHS England, 2014) set forth its ambition to see hospitals become more closely integrated with other forms of care in order to respond to the changing needs of the population and meet the financial challenges. This calls for hospitals to take a system-wide perspective and close working with local partners including primary care, social care and community services. *The Long-Term Plan* (NHS England, 2019) reiterates this objective so that care can be moved outside hospital. As much of the focus has traditionally been on acute care, the government will need to increase funding for primary and community care to achieve this goal. In order to achieve integrated care across the acute and primary sector, the *Long-Term Plan* proposes a reorganisation of current structures so that general practices will join together and form primary care networks, bringing together practices within specific catchment areas of on average 30,000 to 50,000 people. These primary care networks are expected to take proactive measures by identifying people who need support to manage their health. A shared savings scheme will be developed and primary care networks which manage to reduce admissions to Accident and Emergency (A&E), and more general hospital admissions thanks to such proactive measures, will be rewarded. The whole process is expected to be supported thanks to the digitalisation of the NHS which is underway (see Chapter 7). The plan also aims to develop fully-integrated community-based healthcare by developing multidisciplinary teams which include General Practitioners (GPs), pharmacists, district nurses and allied health professionals across the primary care institutions and hospitals (NHS England, 2019). Part of the framework also looks at ensuring enough attention is given to mental health services.

Achieving Parity Between Physical and Mental Healthcare

Until the 1960s, mental health patients were treated in psychiatric hospitals. It was not until the 1959 Mental Health Act that a move towards community-based services was developed. A series of white papers were published: *Better Services for the Mentally Ill* (Department of Health and Social Security, 1975) which encouraged the integration of hospital services, while *Modernising Mental Health Services* (Department of Health, 1998) aimed to address failures in community care and provide extra beds for mental health patients. In 1999, A National Service Framework for Mental Health was established, setting standards in five areas: health promotion, primary care and access to services, services for people with severe mental illness, carers and prevention of suicide. In 2007, a Department of Health report noted significant improvements in terms of mental health provision in the community. A WHO report published the same year also rated mental services in the UK to be the best in Europe (Ham, 2009). On the other hand, services for dealing with dementia did not match this performance.

Nevertheless, budget restrictions have continued to thwart a really effective development of mental health services and an integration of services. The financial crisis has also put increasing pressure on mental health trusts that provide the majority of mental healthcare in the UK. As Gilbert (2016) underlines, funding for mental health has fallen with cuts to these budgets between 2011/12 and 2014/5, whereas many other areas of health, especially acute services for physical healthcare, have experienced rises in funding over the same period. This would seem to contradict the NHS's 2014 pledge to achieve parity between mental and physical health by 2020 (NHS England, 2014; Gilbert, 2016).

An independent Mental Health Taskforce underlined the need to improve crisis and acute care for mental health patients. Commissioners were said not to be using available funding for the purposes intended: they tended to focus on tackling acute sector deficits rather than those in the mental health sector. It would seem that payment systems also make managing mental health difficult because providers are paid through block contracts, which are difficult to adjust to meet demand and are more exposed to cuts across all areas of mental health. Such financial pressures have led to the reduction of mental health staff by around 40% (Gilbert, 2016). Staff shortages have meant that mental health institutions are unable to meet the NHS England standards introduced in 2016. Around a quarter of Clinical Commissioning Groups (CCGs) failed to meet the targets. Therefore, despite the impetus to join-up physical and mental health, as outlined in the *Five Year Forward* report (NHS England, 2014), there would seem to be major difficulties in providing the necessary basis for a joined-up approach. Nevertheless, in the *Long-Term Plan*, NHS England has again promised more investment in order to join-up physical and mental health (NHS England, 2019). It underlines that often those living with a serious mental illness are also suffering from a physical long-term condition such as asthma, diabetes, obesity, chronic obstructive pulmonary disease or cardiovascular disease. The *Long-Term Plan* has committed to increasing joint mental and physical health checks for an additional 110, 000 people per year (NHS England, 2019).

Joining-Up Health and Social Care

Another priority set forth in the *Five Year Forward* report (NHS England, 2014) and reiterated in the *Long-Term Plan* (NHS England, 2019) is the integration of health and social care. While healthcare remains free at the point of use, social care has become largely needs and means tested. Income and assets must be very low to receive free care in a residential or nursing home. More than half of social care is paid for privately. However, the significant social, demographic and technological changes have put increasing pressure on social care. People are able to live longer with chronic diseases thanks to advancements in healthcare, but this also means that there are more elderly people living with multiple conditions which require both health and social care. It is in this way that the dividing line between health and social care has become increasing blurred and complex to govern. A number of associations, and notably the King's Fund, have called for a new settlement in health and social care. A recent enquiry by this association underlined how health and social care need to be aligned because healthcare remains largely free at the point of use, whereas social care is still widely needs and means tested, which creates inequalities. This has led to increasing calls for a single ring-fenced budget for both health and social care. However, a more coherent funding system needs to be phased in at the same time. The Association of Directors of Adult Social Services (ADASS) carried out a survey to which 95% of councils responded and underlined that the current system of social care was 'unsustainable' (ADASS, 2014). The Local Government Association (LGA, 2014) reported a £1.9 billion gap for adult social care (LGA, 2014). Sir Merrick Cockell, former chairman of the LGA lamented that:

Too many older people are being let down by a broken system which leaves them languishing in hospital beds while they wait for an alternative, or consigned to residential care because we lack the capacity to help them live independently (National Health Executive (NHE), 2014, para. 9).

The situation has not improved since this report was published. An Institute for Fiscal Studies report showed that overall spending on local services by English councils fell by 21% between 2009-10 and 2017-18. The cuts have been uneven across sectors, with spending cuts as great as 50% for planning, development and housing services. Spending on adult care was protected to some extent by councils but still fell by 5% between 2009–10 and 2017–18 (Amin-Smith & Philips, 2019).

Impetus to join-up health and social care first appeared in the Dilnot report of 2011 after the Dilnot Commission was asked to investigate a fairer deal for the funding of Care and Support (Dilnot, Warner, & Williams, 2011). It called for a complete overhaul of how health and social care should be funded. The report, which argued for the creation of a single, ring-fenced budget for health and social care, has been influential in finding a solution for the funding of chronic diseases whilst still maintaining entitlements to healthcare. Despite the clear pressure on health funding, the Commission argued that higher public spending on health and social care would be affordable if it was phased in over a decade. It argued that while this would put increased pressure on funding, GDP would also grow to provide additional funding. It would amount to 11 to 12% of GDP, which is the amount many other European countries pay to cover healthcare alone. An increase in tax and national insurance would be necessary to cover the cost. It should put an end to the current fragmented system of funding and entitlements and make it simpler and fairer to access funds. The cost of care for families would also fall.

However, it would appear that the estimates of the cost in the Dilnot report largely underestimated the amount it would cost to phase in such a system. The continuing process of ageing of the population means that additional funding would be necessary. The initial estimates were that £3 billion would be needed to make social care free for those regarded as having critical or substantial needs, which would then rise to £5 billion by 2025 (Timmins, 2017). According to Nicholas Timmins (2017), despite the Dilnot review and other independent reviews on social care, including one by the Royal Commission and a number of Green and White Papers, no real solution has been found to solve the health and social care dilemma. The essential issue is to what extent funding should come from the private purse.

The health and social care crisis came to a head in the run up to the 2017 general election. There was a public outcry when the Conservative Government put forward a plan to create a 'dementia' or 'death' tax. In order to meet the increasing demands of health and social care, a proposal was made to make elderly people pay for care if assets (including house and savings) were £100,000 or over. This would mean that they would have to sell any residential property over that amount to pay for care. Such a move would in fact deter elderly people or their families from seeking help and inevitably put pressure on hospital and emergency services. It would also probably lead to elderly people simply putting their house in their children's name or offshoring assets (Timmins, 2017). Increasing pressure led to Prime Minister Theresa May revising the initial proposal and suggesting a cap so that pensioners would not have to pay for their own care once their savings and assets came to £100,000. Moreover, elderly people would not have to sell their home in their lifetime, but could borrow and the loan would be deducted from their estate after their death.

The essential problem remains the joining-up of different services. It is very difficult to unite social care and healthcare to deal with the expanding needs in long-term care because there is not one overall body in charge. As the table below illustrates, in most localities long-term care is the responsibility of the Department for Communities and Local Government (DCLG), the Department of Work and Pensions (DWP), the Overseas Development Institute (ODI), the Department of Health (DoH) and the Department for Education (DfE):

One of the essential challenges across the health and social care sectors is the delay in discharge from hospital and ensuring the transfer of care to

Table 1. Leadership in Health and Social Care

Children's social care – local government Adult social care for working age disabled people – local government Adult social care for older people – local government Continuing Healthcare for people with chronic health conditions – NHS Mental health services – NHS and local government Palliative and other long-term care and nursing services –NHS Supporting People funding – DCLG via local government

the community following an acute admission, known as 'bed blocking'. 'Bed blocking' involves the delaying of discharging a patient from hospital for a number of reasons, often caused by the inadequacy of supplying social care (a scarcity of supply of nursing homes, rehabilitation centres or the lack of necessary care in the community). A study by Green, Dorling, Minton, & Pickett (2017) published in the *Journal of Epidemiology and Community Health* found that delayed discharge from hospital in 2015 was associated with increases in mortality. They found evidence to suggest that bed blocking could be associated with up to a fifth of mortality increases. They conclude that reduced quality in performance of the NHS since the austerity measures of 2010 has resulted in such poor outcomes. Elderly people are increasingly in danger of contracting infections the longer they stay in hospital. Admissions are also delayed as a result of bed blocking, which can also result in fatal casualties.

Integrated Models of Care for the Localities

In order to resolve such problems, the *Five Year Forward* publication called for the integration of not only hospital and primary care providers – Primary and Acute Care Systems (or PACs) but also social care (NHS England, 2014). In March 2015, nine sites were selected to pilot a programme of integration between primary and acute care systems. The PACS bring together acute, primary, community, mental health and, in some cases, social care providers. Key difficulties have arisen from the development of sound governance and leadership across providers. Providing new complex contracts has also been very difficult.

The five-year Sustainability and Transformation Plans (STPs) have also been set up to ensure better integration of health and social care in the regions. NHS organisations across the country have been asked to come together to plan for the future of health and care services in their area. The leaders of STPs (mainly from CCGs) have been commissioned to develop new models of care, improve health and wellbeing and efficiency of services. The leaders were asked to identify key priorities in the local area and how they can meet these challenges and also provide a financial balance. This is seen as a move away from the competitive element of the Health and Social Care Act of 2012, which encouraged NHS organisations to compete. They have now been asked to collaborate in a new approach called ‘place-based planning’. It would seem therefore that there has been an ideological shift and that integrated models of care are necessary to meet the needs of the population, with the NHS and social care system working alongside each other. The idea is to enable the new bodies created under the Health and Social Care Act 2012 (local enterprise partnerships, city regions and Health and Wellbeing Boards) to work together. However, the NHS has not really been designed to enable collaboration between organisations, so it is quite a challenge to achieve co-ordination.

NHS England plans to transform the STPs into Accountable Care Organisations (ACOs) for the integration of Health and Social Care. While ACOs originate from the US and the Obamacare reform, the proposal is somewhat different in the UK. Accountable care is actually the new buzz word for Integrated Care. The implementation of ACOs would involve NHS providers, the local authority and other health providers in localities co-managing a fixed budget to administer the health needs of the local population (Department of Health, 2017). The aim of the ACO is to establish a co-ordinated approach to the provision of health and social care. Accountable care has already started to operate within the current legal framework. It has taken several forms as Table 2 shows.

Table 2. Forms of Accountable Care

• **Accountable care partnerships** (ACPs) are alliances of NHS providers that work together to deliver care by agreeing to collaborate rather than compete. These providers include hospitals, community services, mental health services and GPs. Social care and independent and third sector providers may also be involved.
• **Accountable care organisations** (ACOs) are a more formal version of an ACP that may result when NHS providers agree to merge to create a single organisation or when commissioners use competitive procurement to invite bids from organisations capable of taking on a contract to deliver services to a defined population.
• **Accountable care systems** (ACSs) have evolved from STPs and take the lead in planning and commissioning care for their populations and providing system leadership. They bring together NHS providers and commissioners and local authorities to work in partnership in improving health and care in their area.

Source: Ham, 2018a

ACPs were actually implemented as part of the Greater Manchester and Surrey Heartlands government devolution programme. ACOs are currently being negotiated by a few localities. ACSs have already been developed in Blackpool and Fylde Coast; Berkshire West; Buckinghamshire; Dorset; Frimley Health; Bedfordshire, Luton and Milton Keynes; Nottingham and Nottinghamshire; South Yorkshire and Bassetlaw; Surrey Heartlands devolution area; and Greater Manchester devolution area (Ham, 2018a).

However, there is much controversy over the actual implementation. Creating ACOs essentially amounts to allowing commercial, non-NHS bodies, to run health and social services, raising fears of the privatisation of the NHS and the introduction of a US-style health system. The ACOs would be awarded huge contracts to manage and provide health and social care and would essentially be in charge of providing NHS services or contracting them out. Proponents argue that such a shift is essential to deal with the crisis of health and social care and the negative impact it is having on the localities. Ham (2018) claims that accountable care actually takes an opposite route to embracing privatisation and competition because the partners involved in delivering care are all public organisations (the NHS, local government, etc.) and are actually encouraged to collaborate and not compete to provide a better public service. He argues that "The vestiges of market-based reforms remain, but they have taken a back seat as the need for NHS organisations to work together to make decisions on the use of resources has been given higher priority" (Ham, 2018a, para. 48).

Analysis of the effectiveness of these new models of care shows that PACS areas have reported a reduction in emergency admissions to hospitals (Ham, 2018a). Six out of eight ACS areas have also reported reductions in GP referrals and flat A&E attendances. The part of the Nottingham and Nottinghamshire area covered by the Mid-Nottinghamshire PACS have seen reductions in emergency admissions that have contributed to bed reductions at Sherwood Forest Hospitals NHS Foundation Trust. Greater Manchester has reported improved access to GP services, investment in mental health services, and major changes to acute and specialised hospital services.

However, a number of challenges remain. Local leaders will need to invest sufficient time and effort to build collaborative relationships instead of competitive ones which are still currently in place. This will also require support from central government. There is also a need to take an ever more inclusive approach involving a wider range of stakeholders, patients and citizens. The King's Fund think tank gives a cautious approval to the effectiveness of accountable care plans to solve local health problems, even though it believes that it is a laudable approach to meet the growing needs of an ageing population (Ham 2018a). Integrated or accountable care requires long-term solutions, but given the short term approach that has been evident in the delivery of health services since the inception of the NHS, it is questionable whether some localities have the capacity to deliver and to make such long-term commitments, especially in light of fiscal constraints. Since ACOs are meeting with such opposition, accountable care plans will have to be implemented with due respect to the current legal framework.

A PriceWaterhouse Cooper (PWC) study of local provision of health services also underlined some problems which prevent localities from developing the place-based integrated health and care systems recommended by the *Five Year Forward View*. It noted a misalignment between national bodies' remits and the objectives of local systems. It also reported that the number of separate bodies responsible for delivering care often results in duplication and complication of tasks, especially for those tasks carried out by the Department of Health (DH), NHS England (NHSE) and NHS Improvement (NHSI). They also noted an imbalance between political accountability, financial responsibility and operational control. A major concern for service providers interviewed by PWC was the lack of financial security because of the absence of a single organisation which could secure and develop critical resources required over the long-term. Local teams were generally confused over the role of national bodies. They noted a continuing division between health and social care and a separation of roles and functions in this domain. The majority of NHS employees interviewed commented that this was a barrier to delivering local integrated care systems. Only 11% of NHS staff felt that the current system in place could deliver effective integrated services (PWC, 2016).

Timmins (2019) identified a number of requirements in order to develop a truly integrated system of care in each locality:

- develop trust and relationships among and between leadership teams
- establish governance arrangement to support system working
- commit to a shared vision and plans for implementing the vision
- identify people with the right skills and experience to do the work
- communicate and engage with partner organisations, staff and the public
- align commissioning behind the plans of the system
- work towards single regulatory oversight
- plan for system control and financial risk-sharing.

However, many of these key requirements may be absent in localities. The question of integrating health and social services at the local level and its impact on healthcare provision is evident when looking at a specific area of care, Continuing Healthcare (CHC), as illustrated in the following case study.

The Case of Continuing Healthcare (CHC): Challenges to Integrated Care

The allocation of Continuing Healthcare (CHC) is ultimately an attempt to distinguish between health and social care needs. It requires working across the health and social care sector to assess an individual's needs. It is thus relevant to include this specific study of CHC because it illustrates many of the major governance challenges relating to integrated care.

CHC is a package of care funded by the NHS outside the hospital for those who have ongoing healthcare needs. It means that all care is provided free of charge for chronically ill patients in their own home or in a care home, with all expenses paid by the NHS. However, the primary needs of the patients need to be sufficiently high to be eligible for such care. It depends on the complexity of the individual's needs and the intensity and unpredictability of their illness. Indeed, the National Framework underlines that CHC is allocated to individuals aged 18 years and older who have been assessed as having a 'primary health need'. The entire decision making process is person-centred, which means putting the patient's needs first. If the patient meets only some of the criteria, the NHS may still pay for part of the package of support through a 'joint package' of care. The aligning of health and social care funding and prioritising the needs of the patient above financial considerations is at the heart of the Care Act 2014, but also, and more specifically, the National Framework of Continuing Healthcare, revised in 2012 and 2018 (Department of Health 2012, 2018).

The assessing and allocating of CHC has improved in recent years. Until 2007, the separation of healthcare and social care was extremely confusing. The NHS Health and Community Act 1990 shifted care outside the hospital. While this led to improvements in primary care, it also increased means testing for social care. Services became more fragmented and the dividing line between health and social care became blurred. Only a very small number of patients received NHS-funded CHC outside acute care units. Local practitioners (often one senior officer in the Primary Care Trust (PCT)) would take a decision on whether CHC should be granted. Demand for such healthcare rose and a number of complaints to the ombudsman and some landmark legal challenges led to the publishing of the National Continuing Healthcare Framework in 2007. However, the application process was still managed by one practitioner until 2012. Since then, a new National Framework has been introduced to standardise the decision making process and attempt to make it fairer, with decision and support tools and a multidisciplinary team (MDT) responsible for the final evaluation of the CHC applicant.

It is important to underline that a lot is at stake in the CHC process. If someone is found not eligible for CHC, they will have to fund all or part of their care costs: care services and home fees, depending on the income of the individual (National Audit Office, 2017a). The legal framework has been set up by the Department of Health (National Framework for Continuing Healthcare) and sets forth how individuals should be assessed for eligibility with supporting guidance. The Department of Health also sets principles for resolving disputes. CCGs are responsible for organising the evaluation process which determines whether individuals are eligible for CHC. They also decide whether individuals are eligible for NHS-funded nursing care if patients are found not eligible for CHC but need care from a registered nurse (National Audit Office, 2017a). All residents of nursing homes are eligible for NHS-funded nursing care although it usually only covers a fraction of the costs of care in a home.

The process of applying for CHC usually involves an initial screening by medical staff (in hospital or the local community) using a CHC checklist (see figure 1) to identify who might need a full assessment. If clinical staff consider that the individual might be eligible then they will refer him or her to the Continuing Healthcare team at the CCG with supporting evidence for a full assessment to be carried out by an MDT of professionals who should be familiar with the individual's care needs: both clinical staff and social care workers in the community. The MDT will make a recommendation about whether the person is eligible and a panel will then make the final decision on CHC eligibility, looking again at the health domains and four key indicators (unpredictability, intensity, complexity and nature) shown in Figure 1.

Using this checklist, the initial healthcare assessor and then the MDT must examine information on the patient (care home notes, doctor's reports, hospital notes, etc.) and decide how significant the patient's needs are ranging from no needs to priority according to the above domains (behaviour, cognition, etc.). The Checklist threshold is set intentionally low so that a large number of people will be screened and not excluded at the initial state. Priority, Severe or High are given score A, Moderate score B and Low Score C. The

Figure 1. National Framework for NHS Continuing Healthcare and NHS-funded Nursing Care
Source: Department of Health (2012)

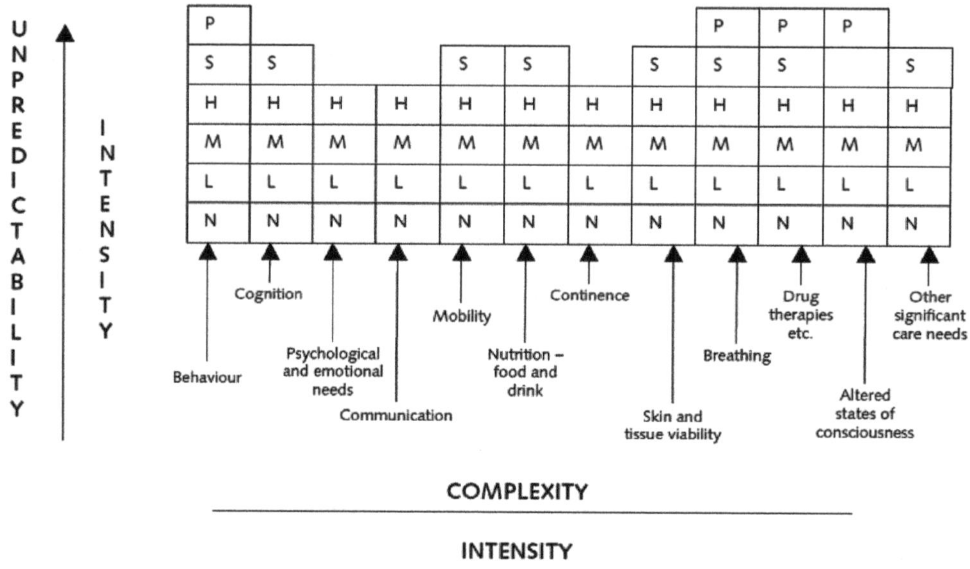

patient will be called to a full assessment if considered to meet any or all of the following:

- Two or more domains with an 'A' descriptor selected
- Five or more domains with a 'B' descriptor selected or one 'A' and four 'Bs'
- An 'A' descriptor selected in any of these domains: Behaviour, Breathing, Drug therapies and Medication, and Altered States of Consciousness_(Department of Health, 2012; Beacon, 2017)

Assessors must also make an overall evaluation of the patient's needs according to the four key indicators: intensity, unpredictability, complexity and nature, after evaluating the domains.

Individuals that have rapidly deteriorating conditions and are approaching end-of-life will be referred immediately and do not require a full assessment. A fast-track pathway tool is then applied by the CHC team to determine eligibility. CCGs must consult with the local authority before making a final decision on a person's eligibility and local authorities should provide advice and assistance to CCGs. The assessment is carried out by one of the following: the CHC team within the CCG of that locality, a CHC team working for several CCGs, a commissioning support unit (CSU), local authority or other organisation.

According to NHS England only about 18% of screenings undertaken led to the person being assessed as eligible for CHC in 2015-16 (National Audit Office, 2017). In 2015-16, almost 160,000 people received, or were assessed as eligible for, CHC funding, at a cost of £3.1 billion (National Audit Office, 2017). CCGs must budget for the costs of CHC from their overall funding allocation (allocated by NHS England). In 2015-16, CHC accounted for about 4% of CCGs' total spending (National Audit Office, 2017).

However, the system of evaluating CHC applicants is very complex because it is ultimately aimed at assessing whether the patient's needs are essentially health or social care needs. An empirical study carried out in 2017 underlined some of the major difficulties in taking an integrated approach in CHC appraisals (Dalingwater, 2018). Thirty-one semi-structured telephone interviews with CHC managers were carried out across England. The CHC managers represented either one single CCG or several CCGs (some CHC teams covered several CCGs). The sample covered all nine regions of England and approximately a third of all CCGs in this country. All CHC teams in England were contacted and invited to participate in the research project but some declined. CHC managers were chosen because they were in the best position to oversee the administration of CHC. The following difficulties in providing a real joined-up approach across the health and social care providers were raised.

A number of CHC managers noted that local authority cuts have had an influence on driving up the number of CHC referrals coming through to the CCG. CHC managers noted that in some localities where budgets have been cut the most, there has been a lot of cost shifting from local authority budgets to health budgets. This varies according to the pressures of local authorities. If the final assessment determines very broadly that the patient's needs are primarily healthcare needs, then the NHS must meet the costs and if they are social needs, the local authority or the individual must bear the burden, which would explain why such cost shifting might take place. As one CHC manager explained:

Local authorities are under funding pressures. (…) I think there are a lot of tactics to manage that whether our local authorities will admit it or not… there is certainly a lot of cost shifting from local authorities into health wherever they can (…) transport services things like that anything which the local authority used to do, it has stopped doing. (CHC Manager, North East).

Approximately a third of the CHC managers interviewed said that some referrals were inappropriate and cases had clearly been put to the NHS because the local authorities consider the care costs to be too high. Austerity cuts on local authorities are therefore clearly having an impact on the NHS:

There is an impact on our funding from the local authority situation at the moment because there is a big push from our local authority colleagues who put people through CHC because they are financially stretched, their funding is having an impact on our funding (CHC Manager, South West).

Nevertheless, this also works the other way: CCGs may be restricting the supply of CHC and deflecting the costs onto the local authorities.

While some CHC managers mentioned that they did succeed in collaborative relations with the local authorities, others underlined significant difficulties:

The largest problem we have is the engagement of our local authority in attending the CHC assessment and trying to create a multidisciplinary team (CHC Manager, South West).

A number of CHC managers explained that the dividing line between health and social care is tricky because the goalposts have changed over the years and this can put added pressure on both health and social care providers. Previously, certain conditions were treated in hospital, but nowadays more and more chronic or mental illnesses are dealt with in the community and classed as social care. This creates clear tensions between health and social practitioners. One CHC manager interviewed was sceptical about the ability of CCGs and local authorities to join forces to provide packages of care such as CHC because of conflicting agendas:

Even if we think about joint relationships and how local authorities and health authorities can work together which of course we are doing strategically more and more so, we are never going to have true joint working because each of you will be delivering against a different agenda (CHC Manager, East).

As mentioned earlier in this chapter, true integrated care requires the coming together of local government services, health organisations and, in some cases, private or third sector partners. Once CHC is granted, CHC teams at the CCG may have to find a suitable care home or set up domiciliary care for the patient. Approximately a quarter of CHC managers interviewed noted that relations with residential or domiciliary care providers were problematic. Owing to a scarcity of supply, care homes tended to drive up prices, making collaboration across sectors complicated. As one CHC manager explained:

We have care homes that are not even coming to see a patient without a thousand pounds a week agree (…) that is a thousand per week with absolutely no clinical justification. So we've got care home organisations and these are mainly national ones as opposed to independent ones that are setting the rate way before they have seen the patient or had anything to do with the patient. That is a huge challenge for us because that doesn't mean that we are establishing anything around a health need, it is actually more to do with the business needing that money (CHC Manager, South West).

Other CHC managers had also met with similar problems:

A key issue that we have is actually trying to find high quality affordable care (…) quality is a key issue…we have an issue regarding capacity and it is a provider's market…increasing hourly rates and head rates…the care homes are very aware that they are driving the market at the moment so from one week to the next, they do try to put up their fees… if they are aware that there are issues around bed pressures, then they will endeavour to raise their weekly rates (CHC Manager, South West).

Soon as you ring up a care home and say I've got a CHC patient, the price just gets escalated, if it is not your own local area (set rate in local areas and local agencies), if they go out of area, so it is not one of our care homes, they just throw what they want on the price (CHC Manager, North East).

In addition, one of the key requirements identified by Timmins (2019) for true integrated care was the need for qualified staff across sectors. Approximately three-quarters of CHC managers underlined in the interviews that staff across primary and secondary healthcare sectors were not always qualified to work towards joint relationships in the provision of care packages:

Indeed, the CHC managers identified inadequacy of trained administrators upstream. Hospital workers or carers in the community were not filling out the CHC referral sheets adequately for example:

You train one raft of staff and then it changes and then you've got people there who don't really know what it [CHC] is. The only way to solve that problem is to include it in some sort of nurse training module (…) It is actually a skill, it is the ability to be able to complete quite a lengthy document and get that information in the document in the right way to enable the commissioners to provide the level of care that's been requested (CHC manager, East of England).

One of the main problems we encounter with referrals is inappropriately filled out checklists by people who have not had any training, or inadequate training (CHC manager, East of England).

The information coming through from the hospital can sometimes be incomplete (CHC Manager, North West).

Collaborations across the acute and primary sectors also seemed complex because of hospitals and CHC teams also working to different agendas and having different priorities. In particular, the hospitals may be anxious to get patients out of hospital into a community setting even if they are not necessarily CHC eligible:

We've noticed in the past few weeks with the pressures on the hospitals that we're getting more and more fast tracks coming through, but only time will tell whether they are accurate fast tracks, or whether it has been a case of 'let's get them out of the hospital (CHC Manager, North West).

Some fast tracks are done as a quick way of getting people out of hospital rather than the correct reason which is that a person has a rapidly deteriorating condition or may be entering a terminal phase. There is some misuse of fast track (CHC Manager, West Midlands).

Sometimes there is not enough information to show why they are end-of-life (…). They seem to be bunched up at weekends and at national holidays like Christmas and Easter (...). If you were cynical, you might think it was a way of clearing beds (…) you suddenly get a flurry of them just before the holiday and then we have to find packages of care for those patients (CHC Manager, North West).

It is evident from the CHC case study that when we are dealing with packages of funding which require joined-up approaches, there are still a large number of challenges to overcome. Referring back to some of the essential components identified by Timmins (2019) for effective integration, it is apparent that many of these are not in place to effectively deliver CHC. A real trust relationship across the health and social care providers in the CHC case is very difficult because providers are working very much to different agendas. NHS health providers are looking to keep costs down and carers in the community may not have the knowledge or the information to assist the CCG administrators in assessing applications for packages of care. The care home providers and domiciliary care providers do not have the same priorities as the CHC teams at the CCGs. The former need to make sufficient profit to continue and they may well take advantage of the lack of demand by driving up prices, whereas the CHC teams need to negotiate adequate prices for their patients. The governance framework is extremely complex because of the multitude of providers. This means that creating a coherent framework and a shared vision faced with so many different priorities and budgets is extremely challenging. Identifying people with the right skills in order to provide a truly integrated approach was also seen to be very problematic. Finally, in most localities the financial risk-sharing which is essential to achieve a truly integrated care system did not see to be in place. This did of course depend on the localities. Some of which had effective integrated care systems which led to better working relations with local authorities, and/or specific agreements to keep costs down with care homes/domiciliary care agencies. In these localities, a joined-up approach was therefore possible and the assessment process much smoother.

Yet the case study of CHC suggests that true joined-up partnerships have a long way to go in England. It looks likely in the future that there may be one ring-fenced budget for health and social care to be managed jointly by health and social care providers. However, conflicting agendas and top-down culture, which still permeate the NHS and local administration, will make this a long and complicated process. Achieving integrated systems is complex though, even in other nations of the UK, such as Scotland, which began the process of integration earlier.

Scotland and Integrated Care

In many ways, Scotland's integrated care system is considered to be the most advanced system in the United Kingdom. In this country, the integration process began as early as 2004 when GPs were encouraged to form Community Health Partnerships (CHPs), which led to the creation of 36 such institutions. The objective of creating such partnerships was to centralise all out-of-hospital care, promote good health and improve workings with local government including social care sectors. In 2014, following on from this process, 31 integration authorities were created across Scotland, replacing CHPs, working across the health and social care sectors. Beyond the previous remits, it also included the integration of emergency hospital care and all hospital care specialities. There had been some successes and failures previously with CHPs (Glasgow being a notable example of failed governance arrangements), so the move to integrated authorities was welcome, giving an important role for local government thanks to legislation (Dayan & Edwards, 2017). The legislation gives much greater powers than the STPs in England or the regional partnership boards in Wales. However, the shift to fully-integrated services is not complete but there are a few localities where the process has been achieved. Ayrshire, stands out as an example where integrated services function well, which has led to reduced bed requirements on inpatient services (Dayan & Edwards, 2017). Scotland has set up a number of indicators for integrated care and measures have been taken to achieve specific targets. The focus is thus not just on hospital care but care across the board and it can lead to more care being provided outside the hospital.

There are a number of similarities in the approaches and challenges met in England and Scotland. Integrated care is rolled out in both countries at sub-regional level with the development of local approaches rather than taking a national or centralised approach. In both countries, there are no arrangements for directly employing staff under one budget. Both are also still finding it challenging to put effective and practical governance arrangements in place to achieve joint working patterns. Nevertheless, the governance framework is clearer in Scotland, whereby chief officers, NHS chief executives and local authority chief executives have control over much of the service planning, funding and delivery (Baylis & Trimble, 2018). Moreover, in Scotland, integration was part of parliamentary debate and resulted in legislation which directs government policy. In England, arrangements are local without any real framework or defined roles, although this allows for flexible approaches to be taken. STPs have been developed around existing legislation, which has meant that managerial rather than statutory processes have directed control and accountability. STPs were created very quickly with no formal discussion or engagement of local communities or frontline staff (Alderwick, Dunn, McKenna, Walsh, & Ham, 2016). They have been slowly evolving into ICSs at an uneven pace. Even so, both Scotland and England have faced difficulties in planning and delivery of integrated services. Even if the mandate is clearer in Scotland, many of the problems encountered by STPs and their equivalent in Wales and Northern Ireland are also encountered in Scotland's ICSs. The clear advantage of the Scottish system is legitimacy thanks to the legal framework but which still allows for flexibility. However, even within a more structured system, it is difficult to assign tasks to partners and to establish effective working relations across the health and social care sectors between providers which have not previously worked together (Baylis & Trimble, 2018). Nevertheless, both systems offer the possibility of pooling funds and thus financial risk-sharing agreements through delegation in Scotland and through the Better Fund system in England (National Audit Office, 2017b). England's system of adopting STPs has perhaps been more complex than Scotland's because the local authority areas do not correspond to the same catchment areas as the CCGs with which they need to join-up, which is not an issue in Scotland. This has led observers to conclude that it may also be difficult for England to learn from Scotland's earlier integration endeavours (Baylis & Trimble, 2018).

CONCLUSION

Whether it be for the English system or other nations of the UK, the same problems of integration seem to be present. The journey towards integration is therefore far from complete. It is so complex because of the need to take approaches which are unique and give consideration to the specific circumstances of each area, matching both local and national agendas and developing effective relationships across health and social sectors. However, the process of integrated care may well be facilitated with the move towards a digitalised NHS which will be examined in the next chapter.

REFERENCES

ADASS. (2014, July 2). *Social care services 'unsustainable*. Retrieved July 7, 2017, from: https://www.adass.org.uk

Alderwick, H., Dunn, P., McKenna, H., Walsh, N., & Ham, C. (2016). *Sustainability and transformation plans in the NHS: How are they being developed in practice?* The King's Fund. Retrieved May 7, 2018, from https://www.kingsfund.org.uk/publications/stps-in-the-nhs

Amin-Smith, N., & Phillips, D. (2019, May). English council funding: What's happened and what's next. *Institute for Fiscal Studies*. Retrieved March 29, 2020, from https://www.ifs.org.uk/uploads/BN250-English-council-funding-whats-happened-and-whats-next.pdf

Baylis, A., & Trimble, A. (2018, June). *Leading across health and social care in Scotland*. The King's Fund. Retrieved February 9, 2020, from https://www.kingsfund.org.uk/sites/default/files/2018-06/Scottish_officers_full_final_0.pdf

Beacon. (2017). *Beacon navigational toolkit – Guide to Continuing Healthcare appeals*. Beacon UK. Retrieved December 9, 2018, from https:// www.beaconchc.co.uk

Boldt, O., Dimson, J., & Kloss, C. (2010). *Supply and demand strategies for lowering spending on hospitals*. McKinsey Publication. Retrieved 31 October 2017, from https://www.mckinsey.com/~/media/mckinsey/dotcom/client_service/healthcare%20systems%20and%20services/health%20international/hi10_lowering_spending_on_hospitals.ashx

Charles, A., Wenzel, L., Kershaw, M., Ham, C., & Walsh, N. (2018). *A year of integrated care systems. Reviewing the journey so far*. The King's Fund.

Cheetham, M., Visram, S., Rushmer, R., Greig, G., Gibson, E., Khazaeli, B., & Wiseman, A. (2017). It is not a quick fix. Structural and contextual issues that affect implementation of integrated health and well-being services: A qualitative study from North East England. *Public Health*, *152*, 99–107. doi:10.1016/j.puhe.2017.07.019 PMID:28881219

Colmorten, E., Clausen, T., & Bengtsson, S. (2004). Providing integrated health and social care for older persons in Denmark. In K. Leichsenring & A. M. Alaszewski (Eds.), *Providing integrated health and social care for older persons* (pp. 139–180). Ashgate.

Dayan, M., & Edwards, N. (2017). *Learning from Scotland's NHS*. Nuffield Trust.

Department of Health. (1998). *Modernising mental health services*. Department of Health.

Department of Health. (2017). *Accountable Care Organisations' consultation on changes to regulations required to facilitate the operation of an NHS Standard Contract (Accountable Care Models)* (Vol. CC17185). HMSO.

Department of Health. (2018). *Decision Support Tool for NHS Continuing Healthcare*. DH.

Department of Health and Social Security. (1975). *Better services for the mentally ill*. HMSO.

Dilnot, A., Warner, N., & Williams, J. (2011). *Fairer care funding: The report of the Commission on Funding of Care and Support*. Crown Copyright.

Gagliardi, A. R., Webster, F., Brouwers, M. C., Baxter, N. N., Finelli, A., & Gallinger, S. (2014). How does context influence collaborative decision making for health services planning, delivery and evaluation? *BMC Health Services Research*, *14*(1), 545. doi:10.118612913-014-0545-x PMID:25407487

Gilbert, H. (2016, March 8). *Bringing together physical and mental health: A new frontier for integrated care*. Kings Fund.

Green, M. A., Dorling, D., Minton, J., & Pickett, K. P. (2017, November). Could the rise in mortality rates since 2015 be explained by changes in the number of delayed discharges of NHS patients? *Journal of Epidemiology and Community Health*, *71*(11), 1068–1071. doi:10.1136/jech-2017-209403 PMID:28970194

Gröne, O., & Garcia-Barbero, M. (2001, June 1). Integrated care: A position paper of the WHO European office for integrated healthcare services. *International Journal of Integrated Care*, *1*(2, e21). Advance online publication. doi:10.5334/ijic.28 PMID:16896400

Ham, C. (2009). *Health policy in Britain* (6th ed.). Palgrave Macmillan. doi:10.1007/978-1-137-01397-2

Ham, C. (2018a, January 18). *Making sense of accountable care*. King's Fund. Retrieved November 13, 2019, from www.kingsfund.org.uk/publications/making-sense-accountable-care

Ham, C. (2018b, February 28). *Making sense of integrated care systems, integrated care partnerships and accountable care organisations in the NHS in England*. The King's Fund. Retrieved November 13, 2019, from https://www.kingsfund.org.uk/publications/making-sense-integrated-care-systems

Leichsenring, K. (2004, July-September). Developing integrated health and social care services for older persons in Europe. *International Journal of Integrated Care*, *4*(3, e10). Advance online publication. doi:10.5334/ijic.107 PMID:16773149

Local Government Association (LGA). (2014, October 31). *Adult social care funding: State of the nation report*. Association of Directors of Adult Social Services. Retrieved October 23, 2017, from https://www.basw.co.uk/resources/adult-social-care-funding-2014-state-nation-report

National Audit Office. (2017a). *Investigation into NHS Continuing Healthcare Funding*. C239 Session 2017–2019. NAO.

National Audit Office. (2017b). *Health and social care integration*. National Audit Office. Retrieved March 9, 2018, from www.nao.org.uk/report/health-and-socialcare-integration/

National Health Executive (NHE). (2014, July 2). *Crisis in adult social care as budgets fall further*. NHE. Retrieved April 20, 2020, from http://www.nationalhealthexecutive.com/News/crisis-in-adult-social-care-as-budgets-fall-further

NHS England Care Quality Commission, Health Education England, Monitor, NHS Trust Development Authority, Public Health England. (2014). *NHS five year forward view*. NHS England. Retrieved March 6, 2018, from www.england.nhs.uk/ourwork/futurenhs

NHS England. (2019). *The NHS Long-Term Plan*. NHS England. Retrieved April 4, 2020, from https://www.longtermplan.nhs.uk/publication/nhs-long-term-plan/

PriceWaterhouseCoopers (PWC). (2016, November). *Redrawing the health and social care architecture*. PWC. Retrieved November 5, 2018, from https://www.pwc.co.uk/government-public-sector/healthcare/assets/health_architecture_FINAL_v2.pdf

Timmins, N. (2017). *Social care: who cares?* King's Fund. Retrieved November 5, 2018, from https://www.kingsfund.org.uk/blog/2017/06/social-care-who-cares

WHO European Office for Integrated Health Care Services. (2001). *Integrated care. Working definition*. WHO.

ENDNOTES

1 The smooth and safe transition of a patient from the hospital to the home.

2 Transmural can be defined as passing or administered through an anatomical wall, but in terms of healthcare it implies the interface between primary and secondary care in medicine. An approach which has proved particularly successful for the treatment of cancer.

Chapter 7
Digital Governance and the NHS

ABSTRACT

The benefits of a fully-digitalised public healthcare system are significant. Digital health is an essential tool in order to improve efficiency, provide coordinated care, and make real health improvements. However, the National Health Service (NHS) has yet to provide a fully digitalised system to patients and providers despite technological advances in recent years. This chapter will thus describe the progress which has already been made in providing remote health services within the NHS. It will also explore problems arising from digitalising health services and the management of health both within the institution and through more informal networks beyond the NHS.

INTRODUCTION

There is a clear recognition from health leaders within the UK that a fully-digitalised NHS is vital for the future of this institution. There are a great number of benefits to integrating digital technology within public health systems. It can provide solutions to many of the challenges raised in this publication: enabling patients to better engage with the health system and healthcare providers, improving efficiency and the co-ordination of care, making real health improvements through technological innovations, providing vital information for patients and providers, etc. While the NHS has used technology in the provision of healthcare for many years, with the first scans

DOI: 10.4018/978-1-7998-3928-6.ch007

and computer technology for administration introduced in the 1970s, the ambition of the Department of Health is that the NHS will be fully-digitalised by 2024. This chapter will explore what the digital governance framework means for the NHS, what advances have already been made and the challenges to achieving a fully digitalised NHS. It will also look more generally at problems arising from digitalising health services and the management of health through more informal networks beyond the NHS.

TOWARDS A NEW DIGITAL GOVERNANCE FRAMEWORK FOR THE NHS

Fully-digitalising health is expected to bring benefits such as improved quality, efficiency and health of the population (Imison, Castle-Clarke, Watson & Edwards, 2016). McKinsey estimates that modernisation, notably through digitalisation, could help save between 7% and 11.5% of funds currently allocated to public healthcare. It can lead to a more active role in managing one's health thanks to information and support provided online (Gretton & Honeyman, 2016). It helps monitor safety and care. It can contribute to making efficiency gains because information is more easily accessible. New medical techniques can help advance medical practice (analytics techniques, machine learning) (Gretton & Honeyman, 2016). It can also contribute towards integrated care.

While digitalisation in the healthcare sector, which implies leveraging digitisation to improve processes, is often seen as a slower process than in other service sectors, such as finance, there has been a digitalisation process in motion to improve the delivery of health services in the UK for many years now. However, it was not until 1992 that a clear digitalisation strategy (or IT strategy) was devised by the NHS Management Executive. Yet the most wide-reaching policy to digitalise across the UK was the National Programme for IT (NPfIT) in 2002. Significant investment, a total of £10 billion, went into this comprehensive health IT programme. The aim was to implement integrated Electronic Patient Records (EPR) systems across the NHS – which could be accessed by 30,000 general practitioners and authorised healthcare professionals in 300 hospitals (Justinia, 2017). However, the NPfIT met with a great number of difficulties and was dismantled in September 2011. The explanation for the failure of the scheme was that it was overly centralised and therefore not sensitive to regional differences or local needs, too prescriptive and offered technical solutions but failed to focus on adaptive change (Castle-Clarke & Hutchings, 2019).

Subsequently, Jeremy Hunt, the Secretary of State for Health, set the objective of a paperless NHS by 2018 (Hunt, 2013). In 2016, Hunt announced further commitments with a budget of four million pounds over the course of the parliament, specifically devoted to digital and technology projects in the NHS (Gretton & Honeyman, 2016). This was also one of the main objectives set forth in the NHS *Five Year Forward View* (NHS England, 2014). Despite these objectives, a paperless NHS has been pushed back time and time again. According to a FOI request carried out by Parliament Street, 94% of NHS trusts were still using handwritten notes for patient record keeping in October 2018 (Parliament Street, 2018). *The Long-Term Plan*, published by NHS England, has promised fully-digitalised secondary care services for the NHS by 2024 (NHS England, 2019).

The Wachter report made specific recommendations to help the move towards the digitalisation of secondary specialist care. To overcome the difficulties in the first attempt to implement a national programme of digitalisation within the NHS, the Wachter advisory group, led by Professor Robert Wachter, recommended that digitalisation be phased in locally rather than rolled out nationally (Department of Health, 2016). In light of the previous failings, the Department of Health also published a policy paper in 2018 entitled *The future of healthcare: our vision for digital, data and technology in health and care* (Department of Health, 2018). It sets forth the government's future plans to ensure a smooth transition to a digital public healthcare system. To achieve the aims of a fully-digitalised NHS, service providers would be guided by four principles: user needs; privacy and security; inter-operability and openness; and inclusion. One of the key requirements was to build a workforce which could support the new digital NHS. It also underlined the importance of equipping the NHS and developing local innovations. In this way it hoped to address some of the failings of the NPfIT (Castle-Clarke & Hutchings, 2019). Finally, the most recent document to set forth the digital ambitions for the NHS is the *Long-Term Plan* (NHS England, 2019). This document reiterates many of the recommendations of the Department of Health's 2018 policy paper. It underlines the need for a digitally-literate workforce, the importance of complying with open standard and it also announces the creation of local health and care records (LHCRs). The LHCRs will provide open application programe interfacers (APIs) so that new software can be created to work with existing systems. The advantage of LHCR is that it can also be used to produce integrated care systems. This would enable data sharing across the health and social care services within a locality (Castle-Clarke & Hutchings, 2019). However, for the moment, most APIs cannot be connected because the system is not ready to support such digital transformations (Castle-Clarke & Hastings, 2019).

Following the Wachter recommendation to phase in digitalisation across the country starting with the most technologically advanced trusts, 17 acute trusts and three ambulance trusts received £10 million under the Global Digital Exemplar (GDE) programme. Those acute trusts who had shown a degree of digital maturity and had already been involved in innovative digital healthcare initiatives were invited to join the programme (Castle-Clarke & Hastings, 2019). However, there is still a long way to go before all trusts become fully-digitalised.

Many trusts have started to embrace the digital age, but some are still struggling with the lack of qualified staff and with specialised technical knowledge. Many trusts report difficulties in finding staff qualified in cyber security, which is a significant issue faced with cyber attacks. Project and programme managers needed in implementing transformational change are also hard to recruit. There is also a lack of experienced senior digital leaders who prefer to accept more lucrative positions in the private sector, with better pay and a clearer career path (Castle-Clarke & Hastings, 2019). Notwithstanding these difficulties, and following the recommendations of the Wachter review, most trusts have a Chief Clinical Information Officer (CCIO) in place, who is considered to be vital to implement the digital transition in hospitals (Castle-Clarke & Hastings, 2019).

But if NHS staff do not have the right training in digital information systems, it may have an adverse effect on their wellbeing and lead to burnout. The Topol Review of 2019 looked at how to ensure that the clinical workforce would be able to work with a fully-digitalised NHS and make use of new technologies including digital medicine and artificial intelligence (Health Education England, 2019a). It also recommends specific training programmes for new healthcare staff. As a result, Health Education England has created the Topol Programme for Digital Fellowships. They are offered to already experienced healthcare professionals (NHS clinical staff including doctors, nurses, allied health professionals, dentists, healthcare scientists, pharmacists and others). The fellows chosen for the programme free up time from their professional activities in order to learn how to design and deliver digital health projects and initiatives in their organisations. A programme of workshops and mentoring is included in the package in order to stimulate and support fellows to be able to lead digital health transformations in their organisations and involve NHS staff in their divisions, and also include patients in the transition (Health Education England, 2019b).

Until 2019, the digital transformation was managed by several bodies, which caused a degree of confusion and inefficiency: NHS England, NHS Digital and the Department of Health and Social Care. Then in 2019, one centralised unit was created to improve co-ordination of the digital transformation: NHSX. Further transformations are planned, with NHSX taking the lead. *The Long-Term Plan* calls for the complete redesign of outpatients services, the reorganisation of pathology and diagnostic imaging services by 2024. However, this needs to take into account that 5.3 million adults still do not use or have access to the Internet (ONS, 2019). Moreover, 4.3 million people reported having no digital skills. These are generally elderly and isolated individuals (75% of those concerned). It may also be problematic for disabled adults to use the Internet, with 23% of them reporting that they do not use the Internet compared to just 6% without any disability (ONS, 2019). This can lead to further exclusion. Indeed, it is often those who have the greatest health needs who are at risk of being excluded from vital health services with the move towards a fully-digital NHS.

Changes need to be more inclusive of users. Digital implementation is not always in line or inclusive of service users. Patients are not always actively involved in the transition. There have also been incidents which have led to mistrust on the part of users, such as the AI/NHS scandal of Google Deepmind. In 2016, the magazine *New Scientist* revealed that DeepMind had accessed confidential health data on NHS patients without patients' permission after partnering with a group of London hospitals run by the Royal Free London NHS Foundation Trust (Hodson, 2016). Despite this, there are some initiatives in place to include users and the general public in the process of digitalisation. INTEROpen, which is an independent action group bringing together individuals, industry and standards organisations, and the Professional Records Standards Body have been working alongside national and local authorities to help accelerate the development of open standards to be used in the health and social care sector.

More still needs to be done to encourage patients to embrace the digital age. In 2019, a patient survey showed that only 15% of patients booked appointments online and 15% reported ordering repeat prescriptions online. The percentage of those having accessed medical records online was even lower; only 4% reported having done so (Castle-Clarke & Hutchings, 2019). Moreover, another issue is training staff to use technical devices.

In comparison to other countries such as Sweden, where patients over the age of 16 all have Patient Accessible Electronic Health Records to allow people and clinicians to access individual health data, the UK is lagging behind (Armstrong, 2020). Natalie Banner, head of the Understanding Patient Data task force based at the Wellcome Trust notes that:

There's a major shift at the central level – but the NHS isn't a single organisation. It's made up of many organisations and there's not nearly enough coherence. Individual trusts – even individual departments within trusts – are entering deals where there's no consistency in the rules or the value of patient data (Armstrong, 2020, para.5).

Moreover, as mentioned in Chapter 2, NHS capital spending remains relatively low compared to other countries. More funding is therefore vital in order to create the necessary infrastructure to have a fully-digital NHS. Indra Joshi, a former Accident and Emergency (A&E) clinician and former head of digital health and AI for NHS England, underlines that even if there is full investment in digital health for the NHS, there needs to be a shake up of the system and support of this fundamental change: "this isn't about throwing money at a problem and at no point is this about replacing doctors – it's about supporting the system so its sustainable while maintaining public and workforce trust." (Armstrong, 2020, para. 18).

Part of the new big NHS project for digitalising the NHS relates to telemedicine and telehealth.

Telemedicine and Telehealth

Beyond the creation of computer records and access to information online, there is a growing market for telemedicine. Telemedicine can be defined as the remote exchange of data between individuals and healthcare professionals. It has been used for example to manage chronic illnesses such as diabetes or heart failure. Clinical signals, video or email consultations can help provide such telemedicine.

Telemedicine was developed in the 1960s and 1970s, but failed to take off because the costs were too high, the images were not of sound enough quality to prove effective and there had not been adequate training (Wallace, 1998; Komaromy, 2001a). However, recent developments have meant that there is renewed interest in telemedicine. It also promotes equal access and the lack of a need for physical presence, which can lead to cost savings. The potential

Figure 1. Timeline of major digital policy developments in healthcare
Source: Castle-Clarke and Hutchings (2019)

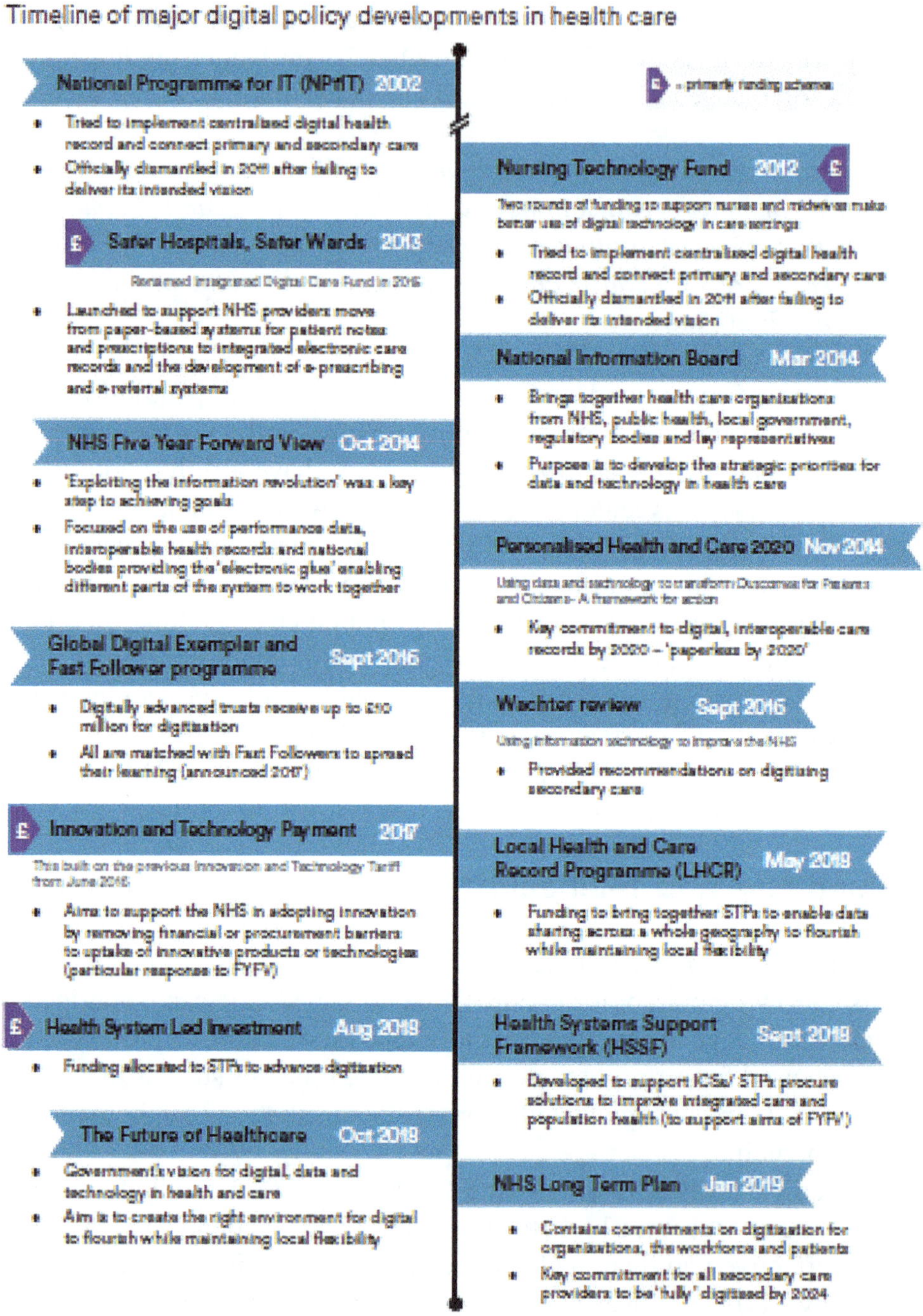

of telemedicine is significant because it means that doctors in hospitals can send images to colleagues in other units to consult for diagnosis. Examples of telemedicine include teleradiology, telepathology, teledermatology, telesurgery, telecare (which refers to technology used to monitor an individual's condition through monitoring their life-style in the home environment) and telerobotics (Lenaghan, 1998; Komaromy, 2001b). In telecare, sensors can be used to detect falls or bed occupancy. Part of the digitalisation of the NHS is the ambition to use digital technology in people's homes, especially so that people with long-term conditions can monitor their health using remote monitoring and digital tools. The Department of Health started to promote the widespread use of telemedicine along with telehealth from the mid-2000s onwards, particularly as regards long-term health intervention. Telehealth includes telemedicine and remote non-clinical services such as provider training, administrative meetings and medical education.

In 2012 a literature review of the effectiveness of such technologies, published in the *British Medical Journal*, underlined that the effects of telehealth on secondary healthcare use for patients with chronic diseases had been tested, but the results were based on very small samples with conflicting results. Nevertheless, the study reported that 65 empirical studies had found that the use of telehealth led to reduced visits to emergency departments, lower hospital admissions and reductions in average length of hospital stay (Steventon et al., 2012). Another study showed that a telehealth intervention using portable devices reduced cost and admissions for people with heart failure. Despite some results finding no significant improvements with the introduction of such technology, the authors concluded that telehealth did seem to help patients to avoid the need for emergency hospital care. Telehealth systems enabled patients to manage their conditions and thus reduce the incidence of acute exacerbations that need emergency admissions. They also reported that telehealth might change people's perception of when they need to seek help and could be useful for professionals who could then have a better idea of when they need to refer or admit patients (Steventon et al., 2012).

In 2010, three large pilot schemes called Whole System Demonstrators (WSD) were rolled out in England to test the efficacy and effectiveness of telehealth and telecare technologies. It was lauded as the largest randomised control trial in the world using three different sites: an urban site (London Borough of Newham), a semi-urban site (Kent) and a rural site (Cornwall). The trial was led by researchers at the Nuffield Trust on 3,230 patients with diabetes, chronic obstructive pulmonary disease or heart failure and conducted over one year. The trial involved giving half the group devices and teaching participants how to monitor their condition at home and transmit this data to healthcare professionals. The other participants received care as normal. A significant drop of 43% of intervention patients admitted to hospital compared with 48% of control patients was reported. There was also a fall in the number of deaths in intervention patients (4.6%) compared to control patients (8.3%) (Steventon et al., 2012).

While the trial showed improvements in those patients using telehealth, it failed to identify cost savings. This appeared to be owing to the fact that while the intervention using technology enabled the reduction in the use of secondary care, the cost of the intervention outweighed the savings from fewer hospital interventions (Steventon et al., 2012). Moreover, the positive outcomes of the large Nuffield study could not all be attributed to technology but to other processes such as more regular clinician contact which was required to conduct readings (Steventon et al., 2012). Nevertheless, the reduced mortality was an important reason to support such interventions and similar technology usage. However, it would seem to depend on the type of intervention, and the authors concluded that it should perhaps be limited to severe diseases (Steventon et al., 2012). Other studies found that telehealth interventions did not seem to have a significant improvement on health, for example for patients with relatively mild asthma (McLean et al., 2010). Although the results of empirical studies have been mixed, technology can play a role in empowering patients and their carers, supporting them to maintain good health and independence. However, maximising the value of telehealth requires people to be actively involved in their care and for it to be built into wider service redesign (Goodwin, 2012; Coulter & Mearns, 2016).

According to a recent survey of chief executives of acute trusts, only a minority currently have systems in place for telehealth (Imison et al., 2016). However, that is not to say that innovation is not happening, particularly in relation to remote consultations and communication.

The recent *NHS Long-Term Plan* has extended the digital ambitions of the NHS, including telehealth. The *Long-Term Plan* announced the creation of a digital NHS front door through an NHS App to provide advice, check symptoms and connect people with healthcare professionals online via video consultations and by telephone. Patients will be offered virtual services alongside face-to-face services by computer or smart phone (NHS England, 2019). The NHS platform has been developed successfully and will continue to evolve. Smart inhalers and remote monitoring of conditions are to be developed. Apps and onlines resources have also been created to support good physical and mental health. In particular, the development of NHS-accredited health apps for patient use regulates and accredits the significant number of apps on the market, such as those designed to help giving up smoking, etc.

The ambition is to provide every patient with digital first primary care, which can save time and travel, to be rolled out over the next five years. In some hospitals, there has been a redesign of outpatient services, online booking and digital appointments. Through the redesign of services, NHS England has set the target of providing a third of all outpatient visits online, which will not only be more convenient and timesaving for patients but also enable the organisation to free up medical and nursing time. It hopes to lead to £1.1 billion a year in savings. While such efficiency savings were not achieved in the past and introduction of technology has been slow to take off, NHS England's most recent report is fairly upbeat about achieving such big technology-driven shifts this time round in outpatient care because there is a strong patient pull to access these services, support from staff, the hardware is available and most people have access through smart phones which was not the case during previous digitalisation processes (NHS England, 2019).

In terms of technology in primary care, NHS England has devoted 45 million pounds over five years to finance the setting up of online consultations. For the moment, uptake is slow but it is hoped that advancements in intuitive, reliable technology and changing expectations from users may increase uptake. In hospital and community care, use is less widespread. Nevertheless, in some specialities virtual clinics have been set up where General Practitioners (GPs) act as an interface and contact consultants and ask for advice. This has been particularly successful in the area of dermatolology. GPs send photos of skin lesions to consultant dermatologists who then make an assessment or arrange a referral. For outpatient care, trusts have also opened virtual clinics. Technicians or nurses collect patient information which is then later reviewed by consultants. In a move to better link up care in homes and hospitals, some monitoring hubs have been introduced whereby clinicians can make assessments or offer advice in order to reduce the number of A&E admissions.

Some GP practices offer appointments online only. For example, *GP at Hand* serves online patients only. Over 75,000 people have *GP at Hand* as their NHS GP, with a 96% satisfaction rate (NHS UK, 2020), which is significant compared to average GP practices sizes of approximately 8,700. Such practices can thus manage a far greater number of patients. The system operates by downloading a Babylon app. The patient can then book an appointment online 24/7 and will be seen within two hours of the time of the appointment. The doctor calls the patient on the app when it is time for the appointment. Via a video consultation, the doctor discusses symptoms and may ask the patient to show him or her things on camera such as a skin rash or perform checks such as feeling glands on the neck. The appointment is recorded so that if the patient needs to be reminded of the doctor's advice, they can review the appointment and see the doctor's notes. Clinical records can also be checked within the application. If face-to-face checks are required, then the patient is given a choice of a number of clinics where they can attend an in-person appointment (NHS UK, 2020). Video consultations and asynchronous communication does not necessarily challenge the fundamental principal of healthcare delivery, but they are creating new models of care. The intention behind offering remote appointments is to improve access between patients and GPs, between GPs and consultants, in order to reduce unnecessary referrals to secondary care, to ensure a better follow-up for outpatients and A&E attendances.

The issue is to what extent patients will engage in online consultations. While uptake has been historically low, in an Ipsos Mori poll 63% of respondents said they would be willing to accept a video consultation with their GP for minor ailments, 55% for ongoing problems or conditions and 43% for immediate or emergency medical advice. A quarter of pollsters over 65 however expressed they would not want a video consultation for any of the aforementioned ailments. There seemed to be a socio-economic difference which was greater than the age variations. More people in higher-income households were willing to use a video consultation in the three scenarios. Overall 71% of households earning over £25,000 per annum were willing to use a video consultation, compared to 54% of those in households earning less than £11,500 and 60% of those earning between £11,500 and £24,999 (Castle-Clarke, 2018). While such changes should improve healthcare delivery, the effects on cost savings are less clear because remote consultations may well increase demand. Kaiser Permanente for example found that offering virtual visits either by telephone or email increased demand from under five million to over ten million, while face-to-face visits remained roughly the same (NHS England, 2019, p. 9).

While many of the health apps have been developed outside the NHS, in order to give advice on reliable ones, the NHS has developped NHS Apps Library which approves health apps. In addition, the Innovation and Technology Tariff reimburses GPs who prescribe an app for people with Chronic Obstructive Pulmonary Disease (COPD). Remote monitoring has also been rolled out for the use of patients to obtain information on blood pressure or blood glucose levels, which is then sent to their healthcare provider or providers. Such monitoring is beneficial because it enables providers to ascertain when a patient is becoming ill and they can then take action quickly. This monitoring has become more widespread thanks to patient apps which enables them to interact with monitoring equipment. This information is vital not only for immediate care purposes but also to provide longitudinal data for research purposes. However, problems may arise if digital tools for self-management are not used correctly, which might be the case for both users and clinicians.

Artificial intelligence (AI), which can be defined as a branch of computer science dealing with the simulation of intelligent behaviour in computers, is only just beginning to play an important role in healthcare delivery. AI could be useful in the future for supporting scientific research in genomics and drug discovery, diagnosis and patient triage, although more developments are necessary. AI might also be used to improve back office functions, scheduling, etc. However, AI does also raise ethical questions. If there is a problem in the system and the patient is harmed it is questionable who should be held responsible for such a failure.

Remote healthcare is thus important to improve access to healthcare services and address patient needs sooner. Technological support can also empower patients to better manage (self-manage) and understand their health condition, adapt behaviour and improve outcomes in the process. However, depending on the process, it may require more significant transformative change. For example, while remote care may not fundamentally change the delivery of care to patients, just the means, genomics presents entirely new treatment options. It can even change the relation between patients and professionals. It also brings the question of ethics into play and the question of limits to what the NHS can reasonably do with new technology given resource constraints. While new developments may add value and better cures, they have to be affordable. Yet while some processes were not available a decade ago, such as Human Genome Sequencing because of the high costs, the cost has been reduced considerably and it is a much more efficient process. A human genome for example can be sequenced in a matter of a few days, which has meant the UK has been able to offer this in the NHS since 2015. Such sequencing can be offered to around 70,000 people with rare diseases and cancer patients. Technology has also helped tailor treatment according to genetics life-style and environmental information, known as ‘precision medicine’. However, precision medicine can be expensive and so treatments tend to be developed for small groups of people.

The most recent Covid-19 pandemic reminds us how much the NHS could benefit from the full- digitalisation of health services and the use of telehealth.

Covid-19 and Digitalisation

Researchers Smith et al. (2020) underline how the Coronvirus (Covid-19) pandemic 2019/2020 reveals just how essential telehealth is in order to deliver care. Using telehealth systems is an effective way of eliminating the risk of cross-contamination and respecting the importance of social distancing. For patients with Covid-19 and/or vulnerable adults, telehealth can provide safe and convenient access to routine care and avoid risks to exposure either in a primary or acute healthcare setting. However, in order to use telehealth effectively, it already needs to be a routine part of the health system. This is already in progress in the UK but not yet fully-operational, as mentioned previously. It requires a significant change in governance patterns, that is in management efforts and a redesign of existing models of care. More generally, telehealth allows patients to navigate the health system and access routine care which is more difficult to provide during an infectious disease outbreak. Telehealth has been used in the past when face-to-face interventions were impossible. In the USA, during the Harvey and Irma hurricanes, private telemedicine companies provided care to victims who had to be relocated from their homes. During the Severe Acute Respiratory Syndrom (SARS) pandemic in 2003, China started to use telehealth and electronic medical systems (Smith et al., 2020).

Despite the potential benefits of telehealth, progress to introduce telehealth systems has been fraught with difficulties in the UK and elsewhere in the world. Uptake has been slow because of a reluctance on the part of clinicians, financial difficulties and the overhaul and reorganisation of health systems that this would imply. The workforce need the skills to be able to switch to such delivery modes. Currently, there is limited telehealth training in medical nursing and health curricula and training. Clinicians also need to be convinced that telehealth is effective, safe and normal (Smith et al., 2020). It needs a wholescale change through all practices, and not just an individual approach, to be effective. Change management strategies are required to support clinicians because telehealth is effectively a disruptive process (Smith et al., 2020). Smith et al. (2020) point to a number of key requirements to fully convert to telehealth: adequate training, telehealth accreditation for health professionals, adequate funding, a redesigning of clinical models of care, stakeholder support, an effective communication and change management strategy and a management system for telehealth services. In practice, it really implies a wholescale reform of governance practices in the UK as mentioned earlier.

Nevertheless, the NHS has shored up their online services amid the coronavirus crisis. The health service in England launched a NHS 111 online tool to provide quick advice on the coronavirus. In the first week over 70,000 people used the service to receive medical information and advice. The NHS 111 service has also referred some patients for a 'drive-through' test in London. This service has enabled residents in each area to get timely advice and reduce pressure on the NHS. Hospitals in England have been encouraged to carry out video consultations when they have the facilities and capacity to do so. These facilities ensure that the NHS can still provide high quality primary care (GP advice and support) at a safe distance despite the Covid-19 crisis. As Juliet Bauer, former NHS England chief digital officer and UK managing director of LIVI states:

Digital presents an important opportunity – stopping the spread of disease whilst increasing NHS capacity, ensuring the NHS can continue to deliver high quality primary care to patients across the UK (Downey, 2020, para. 7).

Such services are in addition to the aforementioned online services which were already in place before the Covid-19 pandemic, which has given more impetus to providing services on a wider scale.

Moreover, the NHS (NHSX notably) is currently working with US tech companies Palantir, Microsoft and Amazon to develop a data platform to inform the Covid-19 response. NHS England and NHS Improvement have joined forces to collate data across the NHS and social care organisations, including the NHS 111 call centre, NHS digital and Public Health England, to harmonise data to have a single and reliable source of information to produce dashboards of information and live metrics. Such information should help the NHS and partner organisations to understand how Covid-19 is spreading, when there will be new strains and how best to mitigate the crisis. However, Privacy International and Open Rights groups have expressed concern that it could be used inappropriately, for example to flag migrants or used as espionage tools. The NHS has also been looking into the possibility of using tools in Google's G Suite family to be able to collect data on hospital responses to Covid-19 in real time which also meets with the same issues (Department of Health and Social Care, 2020). More generally, social media can also be a way in which health practioners provide timely advice to patients, especially during times of health crises.

Social Media and Self-Help Websites

Social media would seem to be the future of healthcare because it enables health providers and stakeholders to communicate with the patient more easily. Social media is instrumental in guiding decisions on healthcare because it can unite and provide support for patients. Patient digital partnerships have sprung up across the globe and the UK is no exception. According to George, Rovniak & Kraschnewski (2013), health professionals have themselves started to use social media in order to help patients, create networks and enhance understanding of issues relating to public health. Doctors' use of social media has risen dramatically from 41% in 2010 to 80% in 2017 (George et al., 2013, ReferralMD, 2017). There are significant opportunities for health professionals to use social media to deepen connections with patients and to reach multiple patients simultaneously.

Patients use all kinds of online sources to seek advice and information. The most common forms of social media are Facebook, Twitter, and YouTube, which are intended to enhance social interaction and collaboration. Blogs, social networks, video and photo-sharing sites, wikis, and other media are also very common. While social media can affect personal lives, they also strongly influence the professional environment. For example, some self-help websites have been instrumental in guiding the provision of healthcare. One such website is *Care to be Different*, set up and run by Angela Sherman after her own parents' experience of the UK care system. Both parents were diagnosed and treated for Parkinson's disease and she had to go through the whole process of applying for Continuing Healthcare (CHC) funding. Her website is a very specialised information resource, which provides practical information about applying for NHS Continuing Healthcare (CHC) funding, but also other care matters. The site provides help and advice for funding, applications and appeals, decisions on care homes and advice on how to prevent earlier discharge from hospital before a proper NHS CHC fund assessment is conducted. Other websites on specific illnesses such as Dementia, Parkinson's disease or Cancer can provide significant guidelines on legislation, help and medication which might even go beyond the scope and knowledge of the local medical professionals administering healthcare to an individual.

However, there may also be significant dangers in the rise of social media in the medical field including questions of privacy, confidentiality, consent, public/private boundaries, professionalism and the risk of misguidance

(George et al., 2013). Nevertheless, social media privacy controls enabling the user to select audiences and restrict public viewing, such as on Facebook and Google+, are somewhat overcoming the privacy risk. Social media also has the power to transform governance through professional connections: Facebook, Twitter, and professional-oriented platforms such as LinkedIn and ResearchGate. Physician-specific networks exist – such as QuantiaMD, Sermo, doximity, and iMedExchange and are also an efficient way of sharing practices and recruiting medical workers. These enable the transfer of ideas, practices and career guidance (George et al., 2013).

Social media has already started to develop as a new form of governance, but the potential for development of health governance is only just beginning. George et al. (2013) for example envisage the possibility of doctors creating a Facebook List or Google+ specifically for patients in order to send information and advice on vaccinations, healthy living, etc. Additionally, the doctor could post short mobile phone videos reaffirming the values they bring to their work, showing a more human side of the clinic and its workers, or encouraging patients who are trying to lose weight. Such tools could also be used by policy makers and health administrators to send out institutional guidelines for digital governance. However, there remain significant challenges in using such means of providing healthcare.

Challenges to the Implementation of Digitalisation

Digitalisation and the development of telemedicine in the cyberworld of the Internet may lead to the control of medical information being removed from medical experts and put in less reliable hands. Security risks such as cyber attacks exist under the widespread provision of telemedicine. Significant encryption methods must be put in place to ensure data security of medical records.

The biggest and most devastating global cyber attack which affected the NHS was the WannaCry hack in May 2017. This led to the shut down of hundreds and thousands of computers around the world while messages came from hackers demanding ransom payments. A third of all hospital trusts in England were affected by the attack and 8% of GP practices. It cost the NHS £92 million because of the lost output of patient care essentially caused by reduced access to information and systems which led to cancelled appointments. The other reason for such a high level of costs was the additional IT support needed to restore data and systems which had been affected by the attack (Department of Health and Social Care, 2018).

Cybermedicine, which can be defined as global medical knowledge and dissemination and access to medical advice and services such as health education, self-help and more general non-clinical information, tends to be even more difficult to control and regulate. The quality of information is also often questionable. It can even create conflicts between sound medical advice provided by health professionals and dubious misleading information (Hardey, 1998; Komaromy, 2001b).

Finally, some would argue that telemedicine also disrupts the relationship between doctors and patients and some face-to-face valuable information may be lost through this form of medical provision. Nevertheless, it is unlikely all physical services will be replaced by digital services because of GPs payments, satisfaction and cultural attitudes towards technology. Elderly people in particular find that a recurrent relationship with an individual face to face is vital.

DIGITALISATION OF OTHER NATIONS OF THE UK

So far much of the analysis has been limited to England. However, it is important to consider digitalisation in the other nations of the UK, notably Scotland, Wales and Northern Ireland. According to a recent Deloitte report, Scotland has made the most progress in terms of training its healthcare providers to use digital devices, whereas Wales has a low level of formal training in place (Deloitte, 2019). This is one of just a few perceivable differences in digital advancement in the three other nations of the UK.

Scotland

The 2018 government publication Digital Health and Care Strategy brings up to date Scotland's advancement in digitalisation in the health sector and sets objectives for the future of healthcare in Scotland (Digital Health and Social Care, 2018). The strategy is described as twofold. First, it aims to enable citizens to better manage their health and wellbeing, support independent living and gain access to services through digital means. It implies that it will make sure citizens can use the tools and technologies available to support health and social care delivery. Second, it will mean putting in place the architectural and information governance necessary for the effective flow of information across the whole care system. There are a number of organisations responsible for making the digital transition possible at both national and local levels in Scotland: The Local Government Digital Office, NHS 24, NHS National Services Scotland, NHS Education for Scotland, the Scottish Social Service Council, the Digital Health & Care Institute, the Scottish Government's Digital Directorate, which includes the CivTech® operation, and the Health & Social Care Alliance. At the local level, local authorities and Integration Authorities, eHealth Leads, clinical champions and TEC leads are also central to implementing digitalisation. In the same way as in England, the Scottish authorities recognise the importance of involving frontline staff and users to ensure such a digital transformation. Similar to the ambitions of NHS England, Scotland is aiming at delivering remote monitoring of long-term conditions through home and mobile health and care monitoring for prevention and supported self-care, maximising use of digital telecare services using smart sensor technology and consumer devices, citizen engagement to enable co-design of products and services to meet the needs of users and wide spread use of video consultations for more convenient access to routine care and specialist support. Chief Digital Officers, Chief Data Officers, Chief Technology Officers, Chief Clinical Information Officers and other similar roles at an executive/board level grade have been created within institutions to ensure the implementation of technology. Given the sparseness of the population and the Highlands, Scotland has had difficulties in connecting citizens to health services, but significant efforts have been employed. Broadband connection has been specially designed to support data-heavy solutions, such as telemedicine, in order to provide adequate care in the country's many rural areas (Digital Health and Social Care, 2018).

Northern Ireland

Northern Ireland's IT strategy has also been similar to other nations of the UK; that is, to organise digital care around the citizen, establish connectivity across Northern Ireland, ensure that citizens have access to healthcare information thanks to a more digitalised system and ensure a fully-digitalised system across the country (Department of Health Northern Ireland, 2016). The objectives of the Department of Health are to modernise health infrastructure and ensure good digital governance. Northern Ireland has been particularly successful in integrating care records thanks to Northern Ireland's Electronic Care Record Programme (NIECR). This system was created in 2013 owing to the need to create a single, web-based, easy-to-use solution. Records include demographics, laboratory and radiology results, medication, diagnoses and clinical correspondence. The NIECR is considered to be very succesful and recorded 700,000 user log ins in 2018 (Deloitte, 2019).

Wales

The Welsh government Digital Health and Social Care strategy for Wales is very much in line with the other nations of the UK: enabling individuals to have more control over their care and improve access to information and services (Welsh government, 2015). They have also adoped a « Once for Wales » strategy which aims at providing all hospitals in Wales with common systems and a common interface called the Welsh Clinical Portal. This provides access to complete patient information from test results to clinical notes. There is no evidence to suggest that digital exclusion is any greater in Wales than the other nations of the UK. However, those living in hilly or sparse areas have been less likely to take up the Internet and, according to recent ONS data, Wales had the lowest proportion of people with all five basic digital skills (66%) and the highest proportion with zero basic digital skills (19%) in 2018 (Deloitte, 2019). By way of comparison, the South East of England scored 86% and 5% respectively in the same domains (ONS, 2019). So even if the strategy in Wales is similar to that of other nations, the uptake by users is more problematic.

Moreover, one of the key components of success in implementing the various digital strategies across the four nations has been how informed and how engaged staff are in the digital strategy. This varies quite considerably across the four nations. According to a Deloitte report, on average 61% of staff felt not at all or rather ill-informed about the NHS digital strategy within their respective organisations. Staff in Wales felt the least informed about digital processes, whereas staff in England were the most informed (see Figure 2) (Deloitte, 2019).

When healthcare providers were asked how well they thought their organisation had advanced in adopting digital techologies, Northern Irish staff felt their organisations were well prepared. NHS Wales scored the lowest with regards to how well the staff viewed the preparedness of their organisation for the digital transformation. In terms of the creation of electronic health records

Figure 2. Healthcare staff views on how informed they are about their organisation's digital strategy
Source: Deloitte (2019)

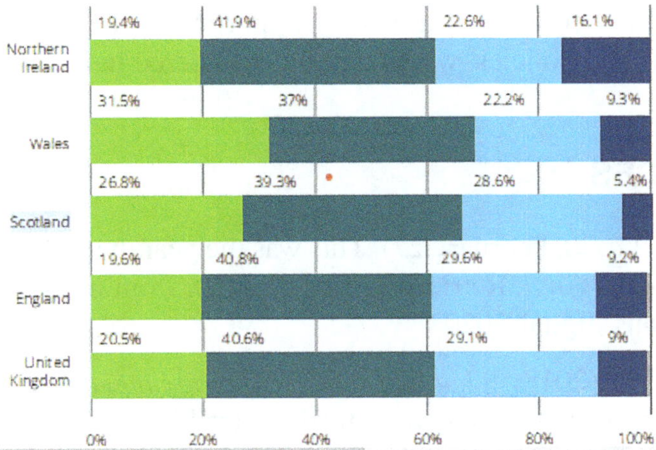

(EHR), Northern Ireland had the highest rate of adoption (100%) followed by Scotland (96%), England (91%) and Wales (78%) (Deloitte, 2019). An essential challenge for Wales is thus to advance with digital change within healthcare institutions and overcome digital exclusion in order to improve the health and wellbeing of the population and reap the benefits of many of the aforementioned advantages of the digital age.

CONCLUSION

In sum, there are significant challenges in providing a fully-digitalised NHS: governance challenges, upskilling requirements, patient inclusion and willingness on the part of the patient to engage in digitalisation, and many security issues. However, there are clear advantages of the move towards a paperless and digital NHS. The most recent Covid-19 pandemic has indeed shown the importance of remote medicine. This is fully supported by key health leaders. As Matt Hancock, Secretary of State for Health and Social Care stated during the King's Fund Digital Health and Care Congress in 2019:

Your banking app works on any device. Updating it is easy and happens in the background. You don't have to migrate the data because the data is in the cloud. There is no technical reason why NHS systems can't work in the same way. The problem is organisational, not technological (Department of Health and Social Care, 2019, para. 19).

Digital health services are also very important in the context of global health systems and policies, which will be considered in the next chapter.

REFERENCES

Armstrong, S. (2020, February 27). This was the year the NHS went digital. What happened? *Wired*. Retrieved April 5, 2020, from https://www.wired.co.uk/article/nhs-digital-2020

Castle-Clarke, S. (2018) *What will new technology mean for the NHS and its patients*. The Health Foundation, Institute for Fiscal Studies, The King's Fund, Nuffield Trust. Retrieved April 6, 2020, from https://www.kingsfund.org.uk/sites/default/files/2018-06/NHS_at_70_what_will_new_technology_mean_for_the_NHS_0.pdf

Castle-Clarke, S., & Hutchings, R. (2019, May). *Achieving a digital NHS. Lessons for national policy from the acute sector*. Nuffield Trust. Retrieved April 5, 2020, from https://www.nuffieldtrust.org.uk/files/2019-05/digital-report-br1902-final.pdf

Coulter, A., & Mearns, B. (2016, 17 August). *Developing care for a changing population: patient engagement and health information technology*. Nuffield Trust. Retrieved April 4, 2020, from https://www.nuffieldtrust.org.uk/publications/developing-care-changing-population-patient-engagement-and-health-information-technolog

Deloitte. (2019, June). *Closing the digital gap: Shaping the future of UK healthcare*. Deloitte Centre for Health Solutions. Retrieved March 29, 2020, from https://www2.deloitte.com/content/dam/Deloitte/uk/Documents/life-sciences-health-care/deloitte-uk-life-sciences-health-care-closing-the-digital-gap.pdf

Department of Health. (2016). *Making IT work: Harnessing the power of health information technology to improve care in England*. National Advisory Group on Health Information Technology in England chaired by Professor Robert Wachter. Retrieved April 10, 2020, from www.gov.uk/government/publications/using-information-technology-to-improve-the-nhs/making-it-work-harnessing-the-power-of-health-information-technology-to-improve-care-in-england

Department of Health and Social Care. (2018, October). *Securing cyber resilience in health and care*. London: Crown. Retrieved April 3, 2020, from https://assets.publishing.service.gov.uk/government/uploads/system/uploads/attachment_data/file/747464/securing-cyber-resilience-in-health-and-care-september-2018-update.pdf

Department of Health and Social Care. (2019, May 23). *Speech, Matt Hancock, Secretary of State for Health and Social Care: Better tech will build better relationships between clinicians and patients*. Retrieved March 29, 2020, from https://www.gov.uk/government/speeches/better-tech-will-build-better-relationships-between-clinicians-and-patients

Department of Health and Social Care. (2020, March 28). *The power of data in a pandemic*. Retrieved April 10, 2020, from https://healthtech.blog.gov.uk/2020/03/28/the-power-of-data-in-a-pandemic/

Department of Health Northern Ireland. (2016). *eHealth and Care Strategy*. Retrieved April 10, 2020, from https://www.health-ni.gov.uk/publications/ehealth-and-care-strategy

Digital Health and Social Care Scotland. (2018, April). *Scotland's digital health and care strategy*. Scottish Government. Retrieved April 4, 2020, from https://www.gov.scot/binaries/content/documents/govscot/publications/strategy-plan/2018/04/scotlands-digital-health-care-strategy-enabling-connecting-empowering/documents/00534657-pdf/00534657-pdf/govscot%3Adocument/00534657.pdf

Downey, D. (2020). GPs urged to go digital to prevent spread of coronavirus. *Digital Health*. Retrieved April 10, 2020, from https://www.digitalhealth.net/2020/03/gps-urged-to-go-digital-to-prevent-spread-of-coronavirus/

George, D. R., Rovniak, L. S., & Kraschnewski, J. L. (2013, September). Dangers and opportunities for social media in medicine. *Clinical Obstetrics and Gynecology*, *56*(3), 453–462. Advance online publication. doi:10.1097/GRF.0b013e318297dc38 PMID:23903375

Goodwin, N. (2012). *Jumping the gun in the telehealth steeplechase*? Retrieved April 1, 2020, from www.kingsfund.org.uk/blog/2012/07/jumping-gun-telehealth-steeplechase

Gretton, C., & Honeyman, M. (2016). *The digital revolution: Eight technologies that will change health and care*. Kings Fund. Retrieved April 2, 2020, from: www.kingsfund.org.uk/publications/articles/eighttechnologies-will-change-health-and-care

Hardey, M. (1998). Doctor in the house: The Internet as a source of lay health knowledge and the challenge to expertise. *Sociology of Health & Illness*, *21*(6), 820–835. doi:10.1111/1467-9566.00185

Health Education England. (2019a, February). *The Toppel Review: Preparing the healthcare force to deliver the digital future*. Retrieved April 2, 2020, from https://topol.hee.nhs.uk/

Health Education England. (2019b). *About the Topol digital fellowship programme*. Retrieved April 2, 2020, from https://topol.hee.nhs.uk/digital-fellowships/

Hodson, H. (2016, April 29). Revealed: Google AI has access to huge haul of NHS patient data. *New Scientist*. Retrieved April 3, 2020, from https://www.newscientist.com/article/2086454-revealed-google-ai-has-access-to-huge-haul-of-nhs-patient-data/

Hunt, J. (2013, January 16). *Jeremy Hunt challenges NHS to go paperless by 2018*. Press release. Department of Health and Social Care. Retrieved April 2, 2020, from www.gov.uk/government/news/jeremy-hunt-challenges-nhs-to-go-paperless-by-2018

Imison, C., Castle-Clarke, S., Watson, R., & Edwards, N. (2016). *Delivering the benefits of digital healthcare*. Nuffield Trust. Retrieved April 2, 2020, from www.nuffieldtrust.org.uk/publications/delivering-benefits-digitalhealth-care

Justinia, T. (2017). The UK's National Programme for IT: Why was it dismantled? *Health Services Management Research*, *30*(1), 2–9. doi:10.1177/0951484816662492 PMID:28166675

Komaromy, C. (2001a). Caring for life: dilemmas in healthcare. In C. Komaromy (Ed.), *Dilemmas in UK healthcare* (pp. 11–20). Open University Press.

Komaromy, C. (2001b). Medical Technology: solving problems or creating dilemmas. In C. Komaromy (Ed.), *Dilemmas in UK healthcare* (pp. 131–159). Open University Press.

Lenaghan, J. (Ed.). (1998). Rethinking IT and health. Institute for Public Policy Research.

McLean, S., Chandler, D., Nurmatov, U., Liu, J., Pagliari, C., Car, J., & Sheikh, A. (2010, October 6). Telehealthcare for asthma. *Cochrane Database of Systematic Reviews*, 10. Retrieved April 5, 2020, from https://www.ncbi.nlm.nih.gov/pubmed/20927763 PMID:20927763

NHS England. (2019). *The NHS long-term plan*. NHS England. Retrieved April 1, 2020, from https://www.longtermplan.nhs.uk/publication/nhs-long-term-plan/

NHS England, Care Quality Commission, Health Education England, Monitor, NHS Trust Development Authority, Public Health England. (2014). *NHS five year forward view*. NHS England. Retrieved January 18, 2018, from: www.england.nhs.uk/ourwork/futurenhs/

NHS UK. (2020). *See an NHS GP in minutes for free*. Retrieved April 1, 2020, from https://www.gpathand.nhs.uk/

ONS. (2019, March 4). *Exploring the UK's digital divide*. ONS. Retrieved March 24, 2020, from https://www.ons.gov.uk/peoplepopulationandcommunity/householdcharacteristics/homeinternetandsocialmediausage/articles/exploringtheuksdigitaldivide/2019-03-04

Parliament Street. (2018, August). *NHS data security: Protecting patient records*. Retrieved March 24, 2020, from http://parliamentstreet.org/wp-content/uploads/2018/08/NHS-Patient-Records-Final.pdf

Referral, M. D. (2017). *30 amazing mobile health technology statistics for today's physician.* Retrieved April 7, 2020, from https://getreferralmd.com/2015/08/mobile-healthcare-technology-statistics/

Smith, A., Thomas, E., Snoswell, C. L., Haydon, H., Mehrotra, A., Clemensen, J., & Caffery, L. (2020). Telehealth for global emergencies: Implications for coronavirus disease 2019 (COVID-19). *Journal of Telemedicine and Telecare*. Retrieved April 5, 2020, from https://europepmc.org/article/pmc/pmc7140977

Steventon, A., Bardsley, M., Billings, J., Dixon, J., Doll, H., Hirani, S., Cartwright, M., Rixon, L., Knapp, M., Henderson, C., Rogers, A., Fitzpatrick, R., Hendy, J., & Newman, S. (2012, June 21). Effect of telehealth on use of secondary care and mortality: Findings from the Whole System Demonstrator cluster randomised trial. *BMJ (Clinical Research Ed.)*, *344*(3), e3874. doi:10.1136/bmj.e3874 PMID:22723612

Wallace, S. (1998). Telemedicine in the NHS for the millennium and beyond. In J. Lenaghan (Ed.), *Rethinking IT and health* (pp. 55–100). Institute for Public Policy Research. doi:10.1136/pgmj.74.878.721

Welsh Government. (n.d.). *A digital health and social care strategy for Wales*. Retrieved April 4, 2020, from https://gov.wales/sites/default/files/publications/2019-03/informed-health-and-care-a-digital-health-and-social-care-strategy-for-wales.pdf

Chapter 8
Managing Public Healthcare Services in an International Economy

ABSTRACT

This chapter differs somewhat in its approach to governance issues compared with the previous chapters as it goes beyond the national framework. In essence, the national and sub-national issues at stake do not quite capture the full picture when considering the future challenges of the provision of public healthcare services in the UK. This chapter looks at healthcare service exchanges across borders. Indeed, there has been a significant expansion of services trade, and in particular health services, which have grown not only thanks to a number of institutional frameworks but also to the support of the British government and health stakeholders. However, there are also a number of risks involved in the international exchange of health services, which can have a significant impact on public healthcare systems.

INTRODUCTION

The international exchange of health services is a rather new development in the UK, but it would seem that the furthering of trade and investment in this sector could have a significant impact on the National Health Service (NHS). The British government and regional authorities are increasingly being warned by civil society and academics alike to bear in mind the risks

DOI: 10.4018/978-1-7998-3928-6.ch008

of the globalisation of health on the British population. Yet limited data exists on the impact of advancing health services across borders with most studies looking at the overall negative effects on public health from trade liberalisation more generally. Health products, notably pharmaceutical goods, are part and parcel of the internationalisation process. However, the impact of the internationalisation of healthcare services, and especially the effects on public health provision, while gaining much media attention, particularly with the negotiation of recent Regional Trade Agreements (RTAs) to free up trade and investment, has remained largely allusive and has been given insufficient attention. The final chapter of this publication will thus examine the issues that have arisen from such processes, how they affect national governance and what might be the implications for public health service provision in Britain.

GLOBALISATION AND PUBLIC HEALTHCARE GOVERNANCE ISSUES

Global Governance

This publication has thus far defined governance in the national and local contexts. However, global governance can also have an impact on the delivery of public health services. Global governance tends to be defined negatively as an absence of hierarchy and a dysfunctional process. Only in the 1990s did the idea of global governance emerge. In 1995, in the first issue of the academic journal *Global Governance*, Lawrence Finkelstein raised the question "What is global governance?" (Finkelstein, 1995, p. 367). He went on to explain that the international system actually lacks central management and control and any clear hierarchy. Therefore, governance was used in the negative sense to refer to the absence of government. Rosenau (1995) describes the anarchic structures of world politics in regards to global governance. It is very difficult to manage, organise and govern the world system of trade and investment in areas such as health because, as Rosenau underlines:

There is no emergent order around which communities and nations are likely to converge. Global governance is the sum of myriad – literally millions of – control mechanisms driven by different histories, goals, structures, and processes (Rosenau, 1995, p. 16).

The vision of a lack of coherence and order in global governance has continued to be upheld by many researchers and described as a "patch-wise institutionalisation of functions of governing beyond the nation state" (Jonsson & Tallberg, 2010).

The need for governance beyond the nation state has been recognised by the vast majority of researchers, policy makers and the like. The reason that many authors give for the need to shore up global governance is the necessity to find solutions to highly complex problems (Altvater, 1999; Hardin, 1999; Peters, 2011). While there is consensus on the need for new governing processes to deal with global issues, there does not seem to be agreement on the nature of such processes. Since the lack of a regulatory framework in an international arena has been established, the next question would be what governance processes could be considered as legitimate or democratic? Legitimacy undoubtedly involves popular consent and clear representation, participation, deliberation, accountability and legality (Braithwaite, 1999; Weiss, 2000; Skogstad, 2005; Bevir, 2010; Considine & Afzal, 2011).

The Commission on global governance describes global governance as:

The sum of the many ways individuals and institutions, public and private, manage their common affairs. It is a continuing process through which conflicting or diverse interests many be accommodated and co-operative action may be taken. (…) At a global level, governance has been viewed primarily as inter-governmental relationships, but it must now be understood as also involving non-governmental organisations (NGOs), citizens' movements, multinational corporations, and the global capitalist market (Commission on Global Governance, 1995, p. 2).

The Commission on Global Governance called for more systemic approaches to deal with global governance issues (Commission on Global Governance, 1995). Ware argues that while global governance is being developed in certain areas, it remains weak in other areas, such as health (Ware, 2006).

The international context of health services makes the question of governing and legitimacy complicated because it requires us to move from the issues raised in the previous chapters of this volume to ever more complex ones. It is necessary not only to consider the difficulties in furthering the international provision of health services, but also how to deal with the wider global harms this might entail.

The Impact of Global Governance on the Health Sector

It is difficult to assess the impact of globalisation on the health sector. There is no established definition of globalisation and researchers have only recently started to reflect on the effects of globalisation on this sector. Lee (2003) underlines that internationalisation processes involve the simple extension of economic activity across national boundaries and the fundamental integration of internationally dispersed activities. This represents a qualitative change and includes the move from a post-industrial or post-Fordist economy to a high tech and ever more internationalised model. Lee (2003) distinguishes between the various processes that can impact on health systems beyond national borders and identifies three key patterns of global change which have affected economic relations.

Figure 1. Globalisation, Trade and Health
Source: Smith et al. (2015)

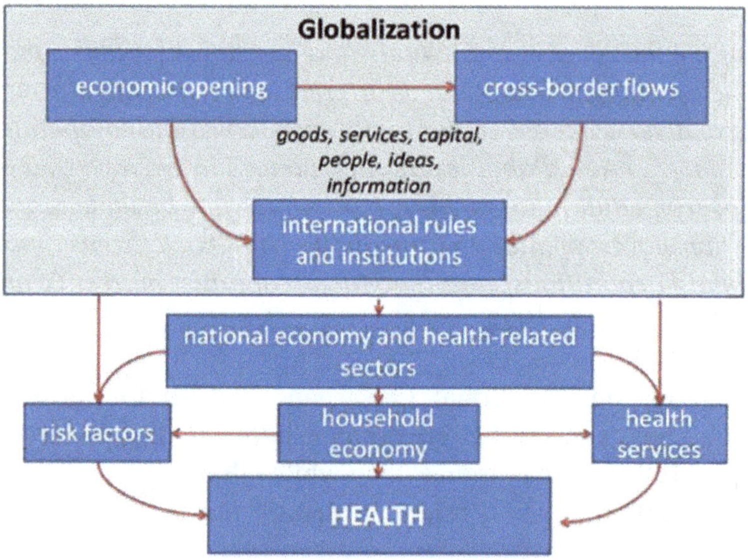

The first is internationalisation, whereby economic entities located in separate territories exchange goods and services. This process has existed ever since the creation of sovereign states in the 15th century. The second process she identifies is liberalisation, whereby states open their borders to economic flows. This process is more recent and supported by international agreements such as the General Agreement on Tariffs and Trade (GATT), General Agreement on Trade in Services (GATS) and the creation of the World Trade Organisation (WTO). Such agreements and associations have tried to free up trade by removing barriers and restrictions to trade and, more recently, to investment. This has also been followed by regional and cross-regional agreements. Finally, the third global change she identifies is globalisation. She refers to Scholte's definition of globalisation:

Processes whereby social relations acquire relatively distanceless and borderless qualities, so that human lives are increasingly played out in the world as a single place (Scholte, 2000, p. 434).

Lee interprets this definition as a fundamental transformation of geography. She underlines that, through this process, patterns of production, exchange and consumption are delinked from territorial space and transcend national borders (Lee, 2003). This transformation has led to the creation of a new geo-economy (Lee, 2003). Such transformations will most certainly impact on human health in general, and on healthcare services in particular, which have been historically constructed along national lines.

The effects of globalisation on the world economy are well documented. Large multinationals play a central role in the creation of wealth across borders and control natural and human resources, capital and investment, core technologies and know-how (Korten, 2001; Lee, 2003). Restructuring and outsourcing has led to what Lee defines as a new geography of winners and losers in the globalisation process (Lee, 2003). Such a process inevitably has important implications for the health sector: basic difficulties in accessing clean water, housing and food. Poverty can lead to inequalities between and within countries and health inequalities. Obviously all such effects cannot be blamed on globalisation, but it is important to put in place effective governance systems to counter such consequences.

As Lee underlines, it is necessary to identify health determinants that are transborder in origin or impact in order to protect public health. While furthering trade and investment in some circumstances can enhance equitable growth, liberalisation has also coincided with a widening of the gap between the rich and the poor and an unequal distribution of income and wealth (Thow & Gleeson, 2017). Global health provision has been part and parcel of the process of furthering trade and investment. However, the public good or public bads (negative externalities) debates are even more relevant in the international arena than at a national level. Transmission of illnesses across borders is a significant health issue. Environmental pollution inevitably has impacts on public health and at some point will call into play health services to deal with such negative externalities. Three main linkages between global trade and domestic health governance can be identified. First, trade brings with it specific risk factors because of the greater flow of goods across borders: diseases related to the changes in food patterns with the internationalisation of food supply, possible harmful substances used on food, etc. Second, trade will also have an impact on domestic supply, including household receipts and therefore public finance available for the provision of healthcare. Finally, there is a direct impact on the exchange of health-related goods and services, such as pharmaceutical and associated technologies, as well as on the mobility of healthcare workers and patients. It is also worth noting that Intellectual Property (IP) protection can lead to a reduction in access to medicines whereas digitalisation of health services can lead to the facilitation and expansion of health exchanges offshore.

Governing health in the international sphere brings with it policy tensions and governance issues (Blouin, Chopra, & Van der Hoeven, 2006). At the macro-level, many of the policy frameworks set forth by the World Health Organisation (WHO), the World Bank and other international organisations have helped put health high up on the policy agenda, but at the same time underline the importance of good investments in health. Investment in health and prudent economics seem to go hand in hand (Lee, 2003).

With the rise of neoliberalism, market forces have significantly influenced the direction of global health governance. The influence of private actors in the global arena has increased significantly. Transnational public-private partnerships tend to have more weight than the traditional multilateral institutions, such as traditional societal and public good values espoused by the WHO. The latter's priorities have tended to depend too much on the influence of private donors (Hawkes, 2011; Missoni 2012). A complex arena of stakeholders raise significant difficulties to co-ordinate and set rules in the new global setting (Missoni, 2012). This is why the WHO has established a framework of engagement with stakeholders with very strict criteria. The problem can be the inter-linkages and involvement between independent and objective institutions. For example, Hardon (2003) argues that the WHO is unduly influenced by companies with vested interests at the expense of equity-focused policies. It also relies on health economists' prescriptions, based principally in US and UK universities or working for the World Bank. For example, the World Health Report (WHR) 2000 was drafted essentially by World Bank economists, health insurance companies, the OECD and private health organisations, but very few health ministry advisers (Ollila & Koivusalo, 2009). The Pan American Health Organization (PAHO) voiced criticisms of the restricted number of circles of policymakers:

It is unacceptable for health policy to be researched and conducted in small, closed circles of consultants and policymakers (…) It is in the very definition of good governance that people have a right to a meaningful say in the decisions that govern their lives (PAHO, WHO & IDRC, 2001, Foreword).

To be fair, international organisations do not all speak with the same voice. While the World Bank and the European Central Bank (ECB) have called for a cap on healthcare spending and encouraged private involvement in the funding of healthcare, the Organisation for Economic Co-operation and Development (OECD) on the other hand has reported that the most efficient health systems are those that are provided on a national basis and provide a universal cover free at the point of use. The OECD has also reported on the underlying weaknesses of the marketisation of health services through the introduction of the purchaser-provider split, decentralisation, payment by results and competition between providers (OECD, 2004). While there is no questioning the expertise in this area, the essential problem would seem to be that, in most countries and indeed in international organisations, health policy making and recommendations have become more and more dominated by the discipline of health economics, which means that other concerns or approaches (such as a rights-based approach) have become less visible.

Conflicts in policy objectives also exist at the micro level and can reside, for example, in the objectives of promoting medical tourism and protecting health services in rural areas. Medical tourism might lead to reducing the supply of health professionals in regions if the former move to urban areas or abroad to meet the demands of healthcare and pursue more profitable activities, such as providing healthcare to foreign-based patients. It is important to ensure that the redirecting of health services to meet the demands of the international market place does not have a negative impact on the provision of acute and primary health services.

Frameworks on human rights and human development help to achieve these aims. Another solution is to carry out health impact assessments of public policies, including trade policies. MacNaughton and Hunt (2011) suggest how such assessments could be carried out: they should bear in mind the human rights normative framework, based on the International Covenant on Economic Social and Cultural Rights, ensuring that human rights treaties are ratified. Taking a rights-based approach, for example, would ensure that governments take the necessary steps to ensure the right to health. An impact assessment should, in theory, provide the state with the methodology to do so and enable governments to choose between policy alternatives to ensure the right to health. A rights-based impact assessment would also ensure that the state is warned if the right to health is likely to be called into question and to take measures to mitigate such effects. Such an assessment may encourage governments to consider alternatives that might more effectively promote equality or correct the reallocation of resources away from rural areas. Finally, such impact assessments would require participation by all stakeholders, so that they can be heard and effectively influence decision making and hopefully achieve transparency. For example, the EU is currently establishing a number of sustainability impact assessments with HR analysis, which do take into account stakeholders' voices.

However, as Lee (2003) underlines, while there is support and a need for evidence-based decisions, this can lead to a plethora of statistics and case studies, which do not necessarily include ethics, moral values and customs. Such normative factors must be borne in mind alongside the evidence-based approach. Moreover, national governments do not always adopt trade policies which are compatible with health objectives. Even if impact assessments are carried out, this might not be sufficient to protect public health. The literature on distributional consequences of public policies and the issues relating to collective action are essential considerations. However, when only a small number of individuals are involved, if interests are diffused or if the potential risks are opaque, then the individuals may have less influence over the policy process. In the case of health, theory would dictate that the policy preferences of those groups that are set to gain, whether they be pharmaceutical companies, health insurance or the like, will prevail. Smaller consumer groups are less well organised and they have less influence. The essential problem is that policymakers and analysts in health and trade hold different views, beliefs and have different agendas. When setting policies for global health, drawing up a clear agenda is not so simple because of the clear imbalance of power in defining policies for global health (Lee, 2003). In the delivery of health services across borders, agendas are set by the WHO, but may sometimes come under the influence of commercial health insurance companies. The effects on the health of the nation will depend on the specific conditions of the health service in the country. The whole framework, channels and intermediate variables must be taken into consideration but causal linkages are very difficult to establish. Health authorities and trade negotiators in national governments are not necessarily working together or at least not most of the time and have little knowledge of one another's expertise. Trade policy reviews do not look very closely at the impact on specific sectors. The original guiding framework of the WTO was negotiated with very little consultation with public health experts and authorities. A significant argument from health associations is that these international trade treaties do not allow policy space or power to enable public health agencies to manage the aforementioned negative externalities that may arise from furthering trade and investment. However, the WTO has tried in recent years to make up for this shortfall in collaboration. For example, a co-authored publication between the WHO and the WTO showed their commitment to working together on global health issues:

As the world becomes increasingly integrated, it becomes less and less possible for different policy areas to be handled independently of each other. The linkage between trade and health has been the focus of much debate: real concerns should be dealt with and any misunderstandings should be clarified based on sound evidence and rigorous analysis. We consider this joint study by the WHO and the WTO Secretariat a useful and timely initiative in this regard. It illustrates that there is much common ground between trade and health. Another important message is that health and trade policymakers can benefit from closer co-operation to ensure coherence between their different areas of responsibilities (WHO/WTO, 2002, p. 1).

It is important to consider the wider effects of trade liberalisation in the health sector and not just the direct effects of increasing trade in goods and services. Researchers and policy analysts, including at the World Bank and the OECD, have underlined the costs of trade liberalisation if supportive policies are not put in place, such as the creation and destruction of employment and increases in wage inequality because of the effects of increasing demand for skilled labour at the expense of low skills. General inequalities can indeed produce health and social inequities. Such evidence is supported at an international level by the work of the Commission on the Social Determinants of Health (CSDH) which shows how health and illness follow a social gradient: the lower the socio-economic position, the worse the health (Weiss, 2015). However, the Commission also argues that much of the imbalance can be avoided by practical and equitable social and economic public policy measures. In order to address inequities, it is important to support a strong public sector which is adequately financed, with effective governance, strong national policy space and support for civil society (Weiss, 2015).

Bearing in mind these complexities of global health governance, which inevitably influence the provision of public health services at the national level, the next section will turn more specifically to understanding the nature of health services, their weight in global trade and investment and the inherent difficulties in trading health services.

INTERNATIONALISATION OF HEALTH SERVICES

What Is Trade in Health Services?

Health services trade is complicated to define, but given a quite restricted definition by the WTO Central Product Classification:

Health services include hospital services (i.e. health services delivered under the supervision of doctors) and other health services (i.e. ambulance services and residential health facilities). It does not include medical and dental services, veterinary services and the services provided by nurses, midwives etc., which are grouped separately under "professional services" (WTO, 2020)

Some essential professional healthcare services are excluded from the nomenclature. For this reason, when dealing with the internationalisation of public health services through trade and investment, our analysis will be broader to incorporate both health services as defined by the WTO and professional health services.

It is very difficult to estimate trade and investment in health services because it is often accounted for in other more general posts: tourism, telecommunications, etc. We can broaden the definition of health services to include information exchange, drugs availability, medical equipment, air fares, accommodation, foreign holidaymakers who use medical centres, business travellers, students, etc. Medical tourism is not accounted for separately in national accounts because it is almost impossible to estimate. The only figures that exist are those provided by the IMF Balance of Payments Statistics Yearbook on health-related travel (Reisman, 2014).

Basically trade in health services works along the same lines as general services across borders through four modes of supply: cross border supply (remote delivery of services through digital health services), consumption abroad (often referred to as health tourism, whereby domestic consumers or patients travel to another country to receive health services), commercial presence (when a foreign service provider establishes a presence in the host country to supply services) and finally the movement of natural persons (the movement of health professionals to supply healthcare in a foreign country, but on a temporary basis).

Global Trade and Investment in Health Services

International trade in health services has been expanding in recent years to represent a major source of growth worldwide. An increasing number of health professionals are moving to other countries, whether on a temporary or permanent basis, to earn higher wages or to enjoy better working conditions. Foreign Direct Investment (FDI) from hospital operators and health insurance companies is on the rise. There is also a move to attract health consumers from other countries. Figures are hard to come by because most national statistics combine figures for health services with professional services or health and pharmaceutical products. However, the OECD produced a breakdown of health services and professional services linked to health in its *Health at a Glance* publication. Total exports of health related travel expenditure and other health services amounted to around USD 6.9 billion in 2011 (OECD, 2015).

Figure 2. Health Related Exports (millions of dollars)
Source: OECD (2015); Smith et al. (2015)

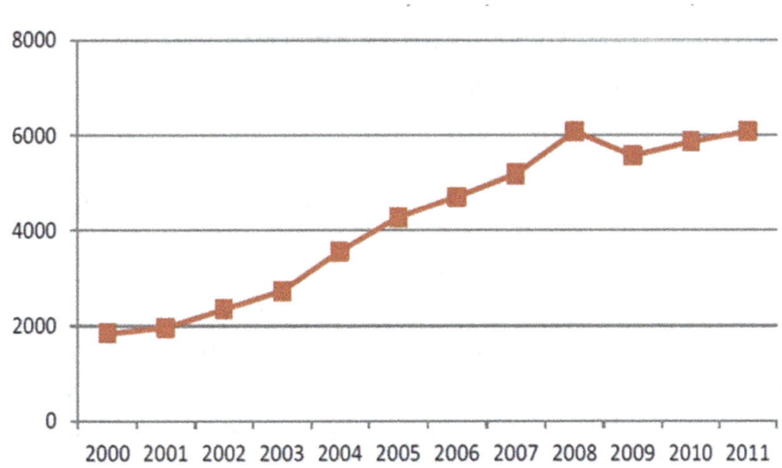

The Private Market for Healthcare in Britain: Inbound and Outbound Trade and Investment

The International Passenger Survey reported that 144,000 UK citizens and permanent residents paid for treatment abroad in 2017. In addition, over 50,000 foreigners travelled to the UK for medical care in the same year (ONS, 2019). One third of outbound medical tourism from the UK was for cosmetic tourism. In Britain, inbound medical tourism is estimated to be greater than the value of outbound medical tourism. This is because the UK represents a very important regional market for in vitro fertilisation. The exchange of care in Europe is important. At least 50,000 UK patients pay for private care in EU. Health tourism is not just an investment good, but is increasingly a luxury consumer durable. As healthcare demands rise worldwide, healthcare is evolving from targets for remedy and survival to something much more sophisticated. There is also an increasing market for healthcare in Asia owing to the rise of the middle classes. It is predicted that there will be a rise in the size of the middle classes from 1.8 billion people in 2009 to 4.9 billion people by 2030. So much of the growth will come not from North America but from Asia. The global demand from the middle classes is expected to grow from US$21 trillion in 2009 to US$56 trillion in 2030 (Reisman, 2014).

Trade in health services tends to take place in the private market for medical travel to have dental implants, orthodontic dentistry, bariatric surgery, aesthetic surgery, skin lightening, rhinoplasty, botox, liposuction, experimental drugs, treatments under trial and in vitro fertilisation (IVF). However, for health services in general, there are a significant number of obstacles to furthering trade and investment.

Non-Tariff Barriers (NTBs) and Complex Issues in Healthcare Supply Over Borders

Indeed, the main issue in health services is reducing non-tariff barriers. The UN broadly defines NTBs or Non-Tariff Measures (NTMs) as:

All policy-related trade costs incurred from production to final consumer, with the exclusion of tariffs. For practical purposes, NTMs are categorised depending on their scope and/or design and are broadly distinguished in technical measures (SPS measures, TBTs and pre-shipment inspections) and non-technical measures. These are further distinguished in hard measures (e.g.

price and quantity control measures), threat measures (e.g. anti-dumping and safeguards) and other measures such as trade-related finance and investment measures (UNCTAD, 2013b).

NTBs in the health sector are quite similar to other NTBs in services. Certain services can be difficult to store or transport, which poses problems for exportation. There is often a need for a high level of person-to-person interaction, which may require a local presence. A number of service providers are small firms, which tend not to be as open to globalisation and less likely to have the financial capacity to export. There are also cultural barriers which can limit demand for imports of services and local restrictions on establishment and operations. Restrictions also depend on the service sector. Barriers are particularly high in professional services trade. For example, economic needs tests may be applied, which means that foreign providers may only enter the market if domestic providers are unable to supply the services and quotas may be established to limit the number of foreign providers. There are often restrictions on commercial establishment. There may be requirements that a certain number of staff should be citizens or permanent residents of that country. Professional services often require government and private sector certification and licensing requirements. These aim to protect consumers but can impede trade and investment. There is indeed still a problem of mutual recognition of professional credentials, non-portability of insurance coverage and a lack of standards for electronic medical records, which can raise barriers to international trade in health services. Finally, concerns about patient privacy and confidentiality issues in distance healthcare delivery have been raised along with difficulties in cross-jurisdictional malpractice liability.

There are also more general obstacles to trading in health services. Communication may be a problem because of the need to speak the language of the destination country. Internationalisation of health services can also be a costly business because not only healthcare professionals are involved, but also capable administrative staff and ancillary staff such as ambulance services (Reisman, 2014). There also has to be an incentive to go abroad for medical procedures. If the price and quality can be matched at home, then patients are unlikely to go abroad for treatment.

Quality is the most important factor when considering undertaking a medical procedure in a foreign country. In an EU poll conducted by Gallup, price was seen to be relevant, but mainly the quality of care and availability of specialists were the main criteria (Reisman, 2014). In Britain, availability of quality specialists and the ability to skip waiting lists were also put forward as important criteria. Having said that, in a treatment abroad medical survey carried out in 2012, 71% of UK patients who sought medical treatment abroad mentioned they had done so to make savings (Reisman, 2014). Reduced labour costs in the recipient countries are the main way that costs are brought down. The length of waiting lists for elective surgery and cancer treatment, for example, described in previous chapters and restrictions on non-urgent treatments, such as IVF, have also been put forward to explain why UK patients might seek private treatment. Given the expense of the treatment, many look to options abroad (Pollard, 2019). However, pricing may be opaque. Problems can arise from cosmetic procedures abroad because of the lack of clear information about the quality of the procedures.

Indeed, it is difficult to retrieve information on malpractice; some countries do not have registered practice listing and, even if they do, bribes may prevent information about malpractice coming to light in public. Birch, Caulfield and Ramakrishnan (2007) found that 60% of plastic surgeons in the UK had had to treat complications from cosmetic procedures performed abroad. Some cosmetic surgery procedures are funded by the public purse. For example, it was estimated by researchers that the mean cost to the NHS of putting right failed cosmetic tourism was £6360 (Miyagi, Auberson, Patel, & Malata, 2012). So, even if such procedures were initially paid for privately, they can have effects on the public purse if corrective surgery is necessary, and this arises mainly because of a lack of accountability in the supply of cross-border healthcare (Reisman, 2014). Training and monitoring of training overseas is often a significant issue. Although some medical schools are benchmarked on international standards, there are difficulties in monitoring international accreditation with different norms and standards.

Limits to competition in the health sector presented by equity, social, cultural and development issues also represent significant barriers because the lives of individuals are at stake. Countries differ greatly on what they consider to be barriers or obstacles to trade. Some argue that the latter are perfectly reasonable parts of domestic regulation (sanitary and phytosanitary standards for example) and protect public interest. Indeed, as Maier de Kruijff, Kainrath, and Tannheimer (2016) argue: "Public Service delivery is deeply rooted in national or even regional perceptions of state and society" (Maier de Kruijff et al., 2016, p. 3). This means that empirical evidence and proposals to support the removing of non-tariff trade barriers must be examined very carefully.

More specifically, there are opportunities but also inherent difficulties in each mode of supply (as described by the WTO trade in services modes of supply):

Mode 1 which involves supplying health services across borders has been helped tremendously by technological progress, which means that services can be supplied remotely where it was previously not feasible. For example, electronic delivery of medical services such as diagnostics and medical transcription, the use of advanced robotics, etc. These kinds of services have the potential to revolutionise the health of populations across the world because they can reach geographically remote populations that otherwise could not benefit from high quality health services. Such health services may also be supplied at a lower cost. However, reallocation of resources may move away from rural healthcare and primary care towards specialisation of profitable export-oriented health services, which can be very detrimental to the health of the particular nation supplying the healthcare.

Mode 2, which is natural persons travelling across borders to receive health services (basically health tourism), involves receiving a variety of treatment from surgery, medical screening, massage and alternative medicine. Benefits of this kind of trade can lead to improvements to the healthcare system for the country receiving foreign patients (the exporting country) and the reduction of healthcare budgets for the country that has sent patients abroad (the importing country). Individuals may also gain from lower healthcare costs and contributions can thus remain steady or fall. However, there is a problem of accountability of quality of care in medical tourism. If the procedure is of poor quality, the home country might then have to provide corrective treatment as mentioned earlier. It is also impossible for some patients to travel if they have certain conditions. International certification of quality standards and a quality international standards procedure would need to be set up. It is also very difficult to find medical insurance coverage under these circumstances. The problem of attracting scarce resources away from rural populations is also a risk. Local prices might rise if there is an increase in demand and could possibly exclude segments of the local population.

Mode 3 involves the establishment of a foreign service provider in a host country. This form of supply can thus generate additional foreign direct investment, help upgrade healthcare infrastructure, create jobs and transfer knowhow and medical expertise. However, these services are likely to be located in highly populated areas, which can increase inequities in healthcare access and the development of a two-tier healthcare system.

Mode 4, which involves the temporary movement of medical staff tends to be more important for developing countries who send service providers abroad. However, there are always restrictions imposed by recipient countries on the number and length of stay. There are significant barriers to this type of supply including visas, work permits, discrimination against foreign providers, non-recognition of foreign qualification and quotas. This is quite different from immigration because it is a temporary supply. The problem for the supply country is a so-called "brain drain".

As Smith et al. underline, the health sector in general has been relatively unaffected by the globalisation process until very recently and this can explain why cross-border trade but also investment is relatively low in this sector (Smith et al., 2015). Historically trade liberalisation involved goods and storable items rather than people. However, advances in technology, e-commerce and web-based medicine have made the exchange of services feasible and the moving of patients and health professionals across borders possible. Transnational corporations have also seized the opportunities of this new growth potential and the increasing fluidity of healthcare facilities, although trade remains predominantly in areas of private health and aesthetical health domains. They do however rely on international governance and, in particular, international agreements in order to further trade and investment, particularly in sensitive areas such as health.

Global Governance of Public Health Services through International Agreements

Multilateral, regional and cross-regional trade deals are intended to increase intra-regional services trade. Trade deals are said to strengthen domestic service sectors by increasing exports, allowing for economies of scale and facilitating knowledge transfer from one country to another. Regional Trade Agreements (RTAs) are particularly popular because they are considered to be easy to negotiate at the local level and often include countries with either geographic and/or cultural proximity. But, at the same time, Free Trade Agreements (FTAs) are no longer confined to trade and investment, but have become significant international regulatory regimes (Henderson et al., 2002, Velut, 2017). In so far as they can impact Sanitary and Phytosanitary Measures (or SPS) and Intellectual Property (IP) protection, the mutual recognition of professional qualifications, and the right to regulate, FTAs are now written as governing frameworks in their own right and can partially control governance in trade of health services.

At the same time, there can be an essential conflict between domestic and foreign interests in international trade agreements. Tensions will undoubtedly ensue from international negotiations, and conflicting international and domestic pressures must be resolved (Putnam, 1988). The new generation trade agreements such as Comprehensive Economic and Trade Agreement (CETA), Transatlantic Trade and Investment Partnership (TTIP) and Trade in Services Agreement (TiSA), perhaps more than previous trade agreements, have encountered significant protest because they represent an unprecedented level of comprehensiveness (Maier de Kruijff et al., 2016). Such debates reveal significant clashes between different regional or cultural regulatory traditions. Stakeholders are not only questioning these new forms of governance, but also the rise of neo-liberal governmentality, which is one way of understanding this new establishment and exercise of political power presented by free trade deals, whereby the concept of governance becomes much broader than the state. Multiple stakeholders are involved because neo-liberal governmentality involves the regulation of populations through multiple institutions and technologies in society (Foucault, 1977-8; Mitchell, 2006; Dalingwater, 2017).

A key problem for the government in the regulation and governance of health policy is the extent to which such overall agreements and globalisation more generally encroach on policy space, which is defined as the freedom, scope and mechanisms of governments to choose, design and implement public policies (Koivulsalo, Schrecker & Labonté, 2009, p. 105).

Trade and Investment Deals: From the Multilateral Approach to Regional Deals.

Trade liberalisation really started to emerge after the post-World War II Bretton Woods Agreements, with the aim of rebuilding the global economy and avoiding further conflict through the creation of an international system for co-operation on trade, finance, and development. The trade aspect was further developed by the signing of the GATT in 1947. The key objective of GATT was to liberalise trade in goods by reducing tariffs, eliminating quantitative restrictions and introducing the principle of non-discrimination between trading partners or between national and non-national products or services (Garcia, 2007; Friel, Hattersley, & Townsend, 2015).

After a series of Uruguay rounds of multilateral trade negotiations in 1994, the GATT then became subsumed into the WTO, with a view to further consolidating trade rules and principles. The main goals of the WTO since its inception have been freer trade by reducing tariffs and customs duties, enhancing transparency, stable investment and stable trading environments and non-discrimination via the most-favoured nation rule (which prohibits the application of discriminatory trading rules between trading partners). The WTO rules have enabled tariffs to be cut significantly and increase flows of goods and services (WTO, 2013, Friel et al. 2015). Since its creation, 24 multilateral trade agreements have thus been created, binding countries on a number of issues. Some of the most significant agreements have been the GATS, Trade Related Aspects of Intellectual Property Rights (TRIPS), Technical Barriers to Trade (TBT), the Agreement on Agriculture, and a dispute settlement system (WTO, 2014; Friel et al., 2015).

However, trade and investment in services have been affected by the failure to remove further barriers and, in particular, the slow progress of the Doha Development Agenda. These were weakened by the 2008 crisis and collapse of financial markets. In Europe, there has thus been an increasing emphasis on Free Trade Agreements (FTAs) and Economic Partnership Agreements (EPAs).

Trade and investment negotiations tend to aim at extending commitments to freeing up trade and to further and deeper negotiations during each round. They often seek to go further than the older multilateral agreements drawn up under the auspices of the WTO. There is an element of path dependency because if previous agreements did not provide protection in specific areas, then it may be difficult to impose these in new ones. Bilateral and investment, but also cross-regional agreements have tended to liberalise further and in this way provide a baseline for freeing up trade in future trade and investment negotiations (Koivusalo et al., 2009).

Since the first multilateral trade agreements, most subsequent ones have included an exception for health, similar to that of Article XX of the General Agreement on Tariffs and Trade which calls for measures 'necessary to protect human, animal or plant life or health'. This clause is considered to uphold the right of national governments to regulate in the public interest, including for health purposes. However, this clause is also open to interpretation and may be contested in the event of a dispute, especially in the area of trade policy where industrialists tend to have a stronger say in the role of the market compared to public health representatives (Thow & Gleeson, 2017).

The GATS agreement was perhaps the first step to providing a common framework for health services: including clauses on health insurance, hospital services, telemedicine, etc. However, it has also been highly criticised for not taking into account the specific nature of health policy in different countries and for transferring governance of public health systems away from national governments. The move towards inclusiveness of services in international trade can be seen as furthering the exchange of health services at the expense of public provision.

European interest groups have campaigned against furthering trade and investment in health services through inclusion in trade deals ever since 2000 during the GATS negotiations. They raised two concerns at that time: that trade liberalisation in health services could have harmful effects on European publicly funded health systems and that this agreement could undermine developing countries' ability to build and maintain publicly funded health services. Both NGOs and public health groups joined the anti-GATS campaign. The main emphasis was on the potential of services negotiations to deregulate essential public services, such as health, by opening them up to private competition. Britain along with other Northern European members (Germany, Scandinavia and the Netherlands) were the most active defenders of health services. From 2002 to 2003 the DG Trade did refine the GATS position by excluding public services from negotiations. DG Trade press releases from 2003 onwards have clearly underlined that "public services" "are fully-safeguarded/defended" and that no commitments have been made in health or education. In addition, Pascal Lamy announced on 5 February 2003 that health and education would be excluded from the EU's service agenda for the Doha Round. A moratorium on health services was also extended to the EU's internal market. From the outset of the Services Directorate within the EU, it was also clear that public healthcare would be excluded from the negotiations (Dalingwater, 2017).

Exclusion of public health services has also been at the heart of more recent trade and investment deals. In the resolution on TiSA, the European Commission promises to introduce a "gold standard" clause to exclude public services from the scope of trade agreements irrespective of how they are supplied, although leaked information in 2015 seemed to suggest that an annex on healthcare might be included to facilitate patients travelling abroad to access health services. After consultation with civil society, the EU's commitment to protecting public services was shored up. While TTIP negotiations have been frozen, Commissioner Malmström confirmed in writing to a UK minister that the NHS would be excluded from negotiations and made the same commitment for the rest of Europe in a letter to the European Social Platform, which is a civil society group. In an EU-US joint Statement on Public Services it was underlined that these trade agreements do not prevent governments from providing or supporting services such as water, education, health and social services. CETA also has a public sector carve-out, which exempts "services supplied in the exercise of governmental authority" from the application of the chapter on trade in public services (Chapter 19), and certain parts of the investment chapter (Chapter 8). Such clauses are thus likely to be negotiated in future trade deals between the UK and principal trading partners post-Brexit.

However, civil society and political leaders are still raising concerns about regulatory loopholes, particularly in relation to the most recent mega trade deals, even if many of these deals have been frozen. Indeed, one of the key issues was the irreversible nature of the privatisation of public services due to inclusion of a negative listing and a "ratchet clause". Under negative listing, trade agreements apply to all areas, unless they are explicitly exempted in the agreement. A negative listing means only exceptions will be listed with no further exceptions after the deal is signed, which could have a significant impact if public services are not included. The negative listing was a key innovation of the CETA agreement for example. Moreover, mega-trade deals, such as the CETA, are described as "living agreements" (European Commission, 2013), which means that more sectors of their economies can be liberalised without having to renegotiate the entire agreement. A "ratchet clause" has been included in the CETA agreement and was planned for TiSA, which means that if a country decides to liberalise the market for a public service then that level of market liberalisation must be maintained and cannot be reversed, i.e. services cannot be brought back into the domain of the state. Maier de Kruijff et al. (2016) underline the essential threat to democratic governance that this implies.

Maier de Kruijff et al. (2016) are concerned that societies may no longer be in a position to reverse negative decisions due to inadequate national policies and will not be able to debate or democratically consult their elected deputies on this issue. Investor protection has also been an issue raised by academics and civil society. The fear is that the Investor State Dispute Settlement (ISDS) provisions in FTAs could enable companies investing in Europe to bypass European jurisdiction and challenge EU government via non-European undemocratic tribunals. This could also apply to the UK after the transition period because such companies could bypass British jurisdiction. This is further reinforced by the fact that the global economy essentially works along Global Value Chains (GVCs), which means that stages of the production process are conducted across different countries, co-ordinated by transnational corporations (TNCs), with significant cross-border trade for inputs and outputs taking place among a variety of networks: affiliates, contractual partners, and arm's-length suppliers with a view to maximising profits (UNCTAD, 2013a; Friel et al., 2015).

While the European Union has carried out impact analyses to gauge the possible positive but also negative impacts of free trade deals, the Faculty of Public Health in the UK argues that inequalities, inequities and general wellbeing tend to be absent from these assessments. They contend that in the 60 pages of the EC's impact assessment of TTIP, while GDP is mentioned 40 times, inequity, inequality and wellbeing are not mentioned at all. The same is true of CETA (Weiss, 2015).

Moreover, leaked documents show the potential for opening up sensitive sectors to trade deals and loopholes. This is the case for TiSA. In 2015, a document entitled "A concept paper on healthcare services within TiSA Negotiations" put forward the case for globalising healthcare services. There is increasing pressure to open up health in such trade agreements. Large US corporations have for example supported TiSA as have insurance groups such as the American Insurance Association and US insurance companies including AIG and Prudential. Some major health and disability insurers such as Liberty Mutual and Metlife have also promoted trade liberalisation through the TiSA agreement. However, analysis of internationalisation has shown that costs could rise, and notably because health insurance premiums would become much more expensive (Public Services International (PSI), 2015).

Nevertheless, there does seem to be an inherent desire in countries worldwide to protect the policy space in the area of healthcare policy formulation and this may explain why efforts have been made to protect healthcare from trade and investment deals. Only 56 of the WTO's 160 Members have made commitments in health services, which represents 35% of its members. Health is the sector in which there are the fewest overall commitments (WTO-World Bank, 2015).

However, there are a number of middle to higher income emerging economies that see health services and particularly health tourism as a way of ensuring foreign exchange earnings and boosting foreign investment and are eager to promote trade and investment in this area. In countries where public services have been significantly liberalised, the fear is that governments may nevertheless be obliged to submit the provision of public services to

Figure 3. Trade in services in developed and developing countries
Source: WTO-World Bank I-TIP Services Database (June 2015)

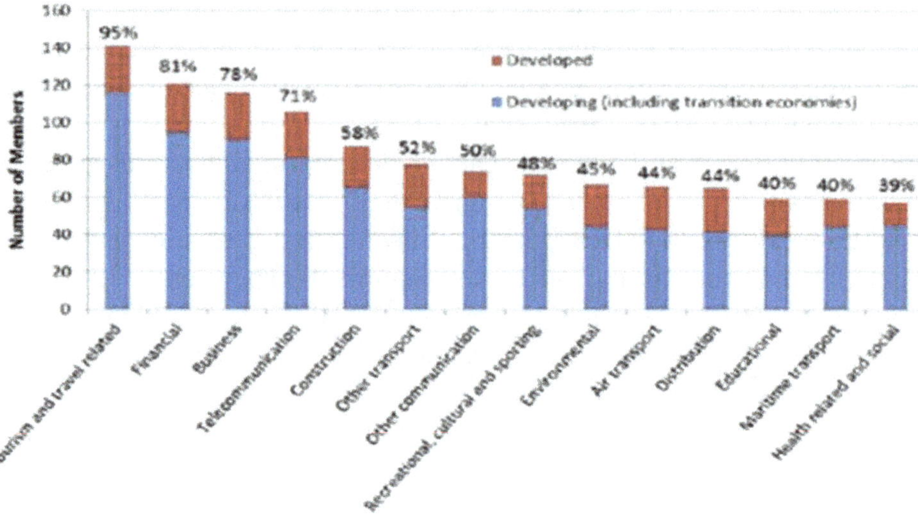

competitive tendering and allow contracts to go to the most effective bidder without taking into consideration service quality.

Indeed, despite such efforts to protect health services, the question is still to what extent public services are in fact protected by such exemption laws given the ever increasing blurring of the public and private domain. In order to assess the level of protection, the major issue is the definition of public services. Rather than using the term public services, most traditional trade agreements exclude activities "associated with the exercise of governmental or official authority" (for example Article I:3 (b) GATS and Article 135(2) of the EC–Chile Agreement). Although they use different terminology, "governmental" and "official" authority, both refer to the function of government in exercising public authority rather than a specific sector. GATS, for example, defines the notion of "governmental authority" as "any service which is supplied neither on a commercial basis, nor in competition with one or more service suppliers", which has been taken up in other agreements (Krajewski, 2011).

It is worth considering the EU's approach because they have thus far been in charge of negotiating trade and investment deals on behalf of the UK. The EU has also taken a hybrid approach in relation to EU law. For example, in public utilities, member states have the right to establish or maintain monopolies. However, the definition of a public utility is nebulous and not defined in EU law. In general, it refers to a service or supply which is considered necessary to the community and usually controlled by a public or private monopoly. This seems to coincide with our understanding of public services or "services of general economic interest" (Krajewski, 2011).

There is also a distinction made between "services of general economic interest" and "non-economic services of general interest", mentioned in the "Reflections Paper" of the EC of February 2011. Non-economic services are referred to as "police and judiciary, prisons, statutory social security schemes, border security, air traffic control, etc.", which can be said to be the same as GATS' definition of "services carried out in the exercise of governmental authority". It also says that it may be possible to "narrow down the scope through a description of the characteristics (services of an economic nature subject to specific services obligations by virtue of a general interest criterion)". Continental European legal doctrine associates public services with those provided by the state or one of its units, divisions or entities. They tend to be provided by an exclusive supplier or a limited number of suppliers regulated by government or government organisations (Krajewski, 2011).

However, it is questionable whether the aforementioned exemptions to public services apply to those sectors that were liberalised in the 1980s and 1990s with the emergence of neoliberal forms of governance. Indeed, the rise in neoliberal policy and practice has led to a significant increase in the privatisation of key government sectors. This is particularly the case in Central and Eastern Europe with the former communist countries developing capitalist economies towards the end of the 1980s. The UK under Margaret Thatcher led the way in Western Europe with a vast project of liberalisation, which seems to have given impetus to other Western European countries, notably France and Germany, to privatise or at least introduce market mechanisms, such as public-private partnerships, albeit on a less significant scale than in the UK. The European Union has also played a role in this drive towards liberalisation of public services with the creation of an internal market and sectoral directives with the aim of freeing up trade and enhancing competition within the European Union (Keune Leschke, & Watt, 2008). This has led to a blurring of notions of public and private and has raised questions as to what extent the state has a role in providing public services. Governance of public services may thus be left to other stakeholders on an international scale.

The threats to public health systems thus tend to be greater for those countries that have significantly liberalised their public services. A distinction therefore needs to be made according to the particular national framework, the development of the latter and how existing and future trade deals may impact on the increasing openness to trade and investment. This author would go further and say that specific legislation in the UK implemented in 2012 has created risks to the future of public health services in an international market.

The NHS, Trade and Investment

While there is potential for private health trade, trading in public services is more complicated both for practical reasons and for ideological ones. Nevertheless, the NHS has made some bilateral contracts for orthopedic surgery in France, Germany and Belgium. While most major surgery will continue to be supplied by the home country, minor surgery is increasingly open and possible in a globalised world. Proponents of advancing trade and investment in services contend that internationalisation of health services can help meet the increasing demand for health services in the world economy and reduce government fiscal constraints. Increased longevity and the ageing generation of the 1960s baby boom years have put significant pressure on health services so there is a need to search for efficiency gains. In addition, there has been significant medical and technological progress, but this has resulted in rising drug and medical device costs and more demanding consumers. Governments are therefore increasingly looking for ways to enhance trade in health services in order to fund rising demand and to keep costs down. It is hoped that cross-border healthcare co-operation can lead to significant healthcare innovations. At the same time, provision of medicines, especially through the Internet, but also satellite TV programmes bring with them potential health risks and significant governance issues.

Contracting Out NHS Services Abroad: Opportunities and Risks

The UK will be looking to make trade deals with the rest of the world after leaving the European Union. Healthcare is expected to be hit particularly hard by Brexit. The fall in revenue from leaving the EU has been estimated to be significant in the area of public healthcare. If the projected drop in GDP associated with Brexit is taken into consideration, by 2020 healthcare spending per head should amount to around £135 lower than if the UK had remained in the EU (Economic Intelligence Unit, 2016). Even without the Brexit effect, the NHS is facing significant funding pressures. The UK will thus be looking to compensate for the shortfall in revenue and the internationalisation of healthcare is increasingly looking like one of the options.

Technical issues can prevent public health services from being exported abroad or becoming part and parcel of future trade deals. In Britain, healthcare is provided without a user fee. It is effectively free at the point of use, paid for out of social security contributions. Therefore, it is not possible to reimburse the price that would have been charged. However, it has been suggested that the NHS could reimburse the price that was paid abroad despite not being able to take into account the pecuniary value of the patient's entitlement at home. Indeed, neither marginal nor average cost are taken into consideration, so it would be a question of negotiating. It might be possible for foreign suppliers to contract with the NHS according to an agreed value per diagnostic-related group or obtain vouchers which might be used either in the public or private/ international arena. It would be in line with the consumer choice policy which has been developed in the NHS in recent years.

The marketisation of health services has enabled the expansion and commercialisation of healthcare according to Mode 3 of the WTO trade in services framework. Mode 2 of the WTO framework which is the consumption of services abroad has also increased thanks to the increasingly openness of the public sector with marketisation of public services in general and further liberalisation since 2012 with the Health and Social Care Act. This has enabled an increasing flow of patients to use elective health services abroad, which may be unavailable, restricted or subject to a waiting list in Britain. While such health tourism may promote economic growth in the destination country, at the same time it can also give incentives for health workers to move from rural to urban settings as we mentioned in the previous section.

While most major surgery will continue to be supplied by the home country, minor surgery is increasingly open to international opportunities and possible in a globalised world. Faced with budgetary constraints, the British National Health Service will be looking at ways to reduce costs and explore furthering medical interventions abroad. A study concentrating on a subset of common surgeries estimated that the NHS could save between £120 million and £200 million annually by outsourcing some common procedures to India. It would also lead to a reduction in waiting times, one of the key targets in which the UK is currently failing (Lakhani, 2010).

However, Lunt et al. (2011) underscore the potential problems of outsourcing NHS procedures. Patients who receive treatment offshore will take the money with them, possibly from the national health system, which could lead to a spiral of low investment in the national system. The state may then continue to invest less, train less and recruit less because of the outsourcing process. It could mean that taxpayer healthcare funding is transferred from individual patients to a private health system abroad. This might be a result of individual or voucher style systems. Healthcare expenditure in a country contributes to economic development because of many spin-offs, which would diminish if more and more health services are provided overseas. Costs could ensue not only if corrective surgery was necessary, but continuing monitoring and security procedures would also be needed. In addition to contracting out NHS services abroad, there is also concern about the scope for further engagement of NHS practitioners in international private sector health activities.

NHS Practitioners, International Ventures and the Implications for Public Health Service Provision in Britain

Since the Health and Social Care Act came into force in 2012, it is indeed clear that the commercialisation of British health services and the health sector at large has started to open up to international opportunities for trade and investment in healthcare. This has also changed the actual ability to protect public health services under already existing trade deals and notably the WTO's General Agreement on Trade in Services (GATS). GATS is designed to achieve progressively higher levels of liberalisation, but it does provide for protection of public health services. Indeed, as we mentioned previously Article 1.3b of the WTO's General Agreement on Trade in Services (GATS) provides for the following exemption:

(b) services includes any service in any sector except services supplied in the exercise of governmental authority. (WTO, 2000)

Nevertheless, the increased foreign direct investment in private enterprises by public organisations can make the most of the GATS provision. Increased involvement in setting up private health facilities for foreign consumers abroad or in the UK could worsen national residents' access to health services if the best NHS practitioners are concentrating on private sector activity to the detriment of the British population. While it has been argued that the private sector may mobilise additional funds for cash-starved public sectors, it is more likely to fragment healthcare systems and lead to disjointed information and practice because of the provision of two-tier and competing systems between those services provided by the public sector and those provided by the private sector (Allottey, Yasin & Tang, 2012; Missoni, 2012).

It is particularly large and influential healthcare corporations that are able to supply health services, whether it be through inward or outward investment, supported by large healthcare corporations and foreign private investment. A key player in the furthering of trade and investment in public and private healthcare since 2012 and the introduction of the Health and Social Care Act, has been Healthcare UK. Healthcare UK is a joint initiative of the Department of Health (DH), UK Trade and Investment (UKTI) and NHS England. Until 2017, Healthcare UK was nevertheless presented as a separate entity with a website disassociated from the Government website. However, the organisation has now been fully-integrated onto the government's website and described as a joint venture between the Department of Trade and the Department of Health.

Both private healthcare providers and the NHS have thus been involved in healthcare agreements, mainly in countries that are looking to improve the domestic supply of healthcare. Since its creation, Healthcare UK has made over £5bn worth of deals. The key markets are identified as China with 18 healthcare projects, followed by Brazil (11), Saudi Arabia (9) the UAE (7) and India (4). This mainly involved setting up healthcare infrastructure services but also clinical services, digital health and education and training. The providers are private enterprises but also public sector organisations: NHS Trusts, Department of Health arm's-length bodies and academic institutions, working closely with Healthcare UK. The organisation argues that such exchange can strengthen global health by sharing key infrastructures and healthcare in emerging economies and bring revenue back to the UK, which could be spent on public healthcare (Healthcare UK, 2016).

Healthcare UK's principal aim is to increase the UK's share of the growing global healthcare market. They act as "the bridge between international demand for healthcare services, systems and infrastructure and the rich pool of UK know-how and capability in these fields" (Healthcare UK, 2016). They are principally engaged in promoting the UK healthcare sector in overseas markets through seminars, conferences and the setting up of business deals. They promote the UK's "thriving commercial healthcare industry and the world-renowned academic sector" (Healthcare UK, 2016). They also act as an advisory body to NHS institutions and other organisations on political, commercial and cultural issues in order to facilitate market access. They promote five key areas: healthcare infrastructure services, clinical services, digital health, education and training and health systems development.

Healthcare UK promotes the furthering of trade and investment, even within the public health domain, contending that the NHS has been furthering trade in health services ever since the 1970s with the Department of Health's "Exporting the NHS". Such a document was published to respond to requests made to best-performing NHS organisations, such as St Thomas's Hospital, to invest in healthcare in Middle Eastern countries.

Healthcare UK claims that the benefits can accrue back to the British healthcare system, securing over £5 billion for the UK economy, with £235 million reinvested back into the NHS and other public-sector bodies. They admit that the profits may be centralised in London with major London trusts and foundations winning most of the work abroad (King's College Hospital, Moorfields, Guy's & St Thomas's and Great Ormond Street Hospital). However, a few regional players have also been successful (such as Mersey Care and Alder Hey Children's Hospital in Liverpool, Leeds Teaching Hospital and Northumbria Healthcare). Healthcare UK argues that there is scope for expanding outward direct investment and inward investment (receiving foreign patients in these establishments by creating private units) because international demand for better and more efficient healthcare is continually growing with the rise in elderly populations and long-term and chronic illnesses.

The organisation claims that foreign direct investment will enable it to share best practices of an equitable health system with emerging nations. In their preamble to a report entitled "Enhancing the NHS through International Engagement", the organisation argues that such ventures also enable NHS professionals to learn thanks to the challenges of delivering healthcare in different markets. They contend such experiences can provide developmental opportunities for UK staff who can learn new skills and gain transferable experience as well as enhancing the global reputation of the NHS.

Healthcare UK also argues that it identifies and manages the risks of international ventures. The organisation offers advice to NHS trusts engaging in international health transactions. It claims to ensure that the quality of NHS services provided to the British public is not compromised by sharing NHS expertise abroad. However, the series of risks identified in the organisation's manual are mainly concerned with marketing the NHS as a brand name, and externalisation risks, but it does not deal with the reconfiguration of the public health system implied by extending trade and investment within the NHS. Healthcare UK does urge NHS hospital trusts to ensure that they are "effectively able to balance workforce requirements for clinical and managerial delivery outside of the NHS with day to-day requirements for core clinical delivery for the NHS" (Healthcare UK, 2016, p. 32). But from a micro perspective it seems rather ambitious to expect individual organisations (hospital trusts and the like) to be able to estimate the wider risks involved in furthering trade and investment in health services.

Case studies of other countries have shown that an internationalised profit-oriented health system tends to distort the domestic market for healthcare. The US market is a case in point where highly specialised and profitable healthcare has been developed. The market has developed a wide range of exportable specialist medical techniques, devices and highly qualified and specialised personnel, but the national health system remains one of the most inefficient and costly in the developed world (OECD, 2015). Issenberg (2016) shows how the same problem has emerged in Israel, which has developed a haven for medical tourists. The latter enjoy medical treatment far superior to that provided to the average Israeli. For less developed countries the risk is even greater. In West Africa, one of the causes of the disastrous Ebola crisis was the state of domestic hospitals. Many local elites went for treatment abroad and opted out of domestic hospitals, and so the latter became under-funded and dysfunctional. Such examples suggest that concentrating on foreign markets for healthcare provision could lead to a significant under-funding of the domestic system.

Katherine Murphy, chief executive of the Patient's Association in the UK, is concerned about the increasing emphasis in the NHS on profits above health outcomes and care for patients:

At a time of huge upheaval in the health service, when waiting times are rising and trusts are being asked to make £20 billion of efficiency savings, this is another concerning distraction. The priority of the government, hospital trusts and clinicians should be NHS patients (Warrell, 2012, para. 7).

Lunt et al. (2011) have explored the negative externalities of furthering trade and investment in health services on home country health systems. Indeed, a number of distortive effects may arise. Qualified staff may divert their attentions to health export services that have better pay and facilities, which diminishes services and facilities in the home country and can perpetuate inequalities. Education and training may be provided by the home country at significant costs, but outward investment through personnel practicing abroad would benefit the overseas country. Free trade agreements could further this tendency towards the internationalisation of healthcare.

CONCLUSION

While the increase in exchanges across the globe has the potential to increase and improve the supply of health services worldwide, a lack of global governance mechanisms to protect health on an international level, and failure to take into account the risks to public health of internationalisation may be highly detrimental to the health of all nations. There would seem to be a number of key risks in furthering trade in health services, whether it be in the public or private domain, such as a resulting two-tier health system, disincentives for practitioners to engage in the public sector and an inequitable access to healthcare. The reconfiguration of the public health system in Britain and recent legislation to open up public health services to the private sector have made this country even more vulnerable to such risks. While it may appear that public services are protected or have carve-outs in free trade agreements, the reality is that said services are still at risk because of current legislation which enables private and public health providers alike to further trade and investment largely unheeded. The biggest risk is the extension of private healthcare and the crowding out of investment in the public sector.

REFERENCES

Allottey, P., Yasin, S., & Tang, S. (2012). Universal coverage in an era of privatization: Can we guarantee health for all? *BMC Public Health, 12*(S1). doi:10.1186/1471-2458-12-S1-S1 PMID:22992275

Altvater, E. (1999). The democratic order, economic globalization, and ecological restrictions: on the relation of material and formal democracy. In I. Shapiro & C. Hacker-Cordón (Eds.), *Democracy's Edges* (pp. 41–62). Cambridge University Press. doi:10.1017/CBO9780511586361.005

Bevir, M. (2010). *Democratic Governance.* Princeton University Press. doi:10.1515/9781400836857

Birch, J., Caulfield, R., & Ramakrishnan, V. (2007). The complications of 'cosmetic tourism': An avoidable burden on the NHS. *Journal of Plastic, Reconstructive & Aesthetic Surgery; JPRAS, 60*(9), 1075–1077. doi:10.1016/j.bjps.2007.03.030 PMID:17482899

Blouin, C., Chopra, M., & van der Hoeven, R. (2009). Trade and social determinants of health. *Lancet, 373*(9662), 502–507. doi:10.1016/S0140-6736(08)61777-8 PMID:19167058

Braithwaite, J. (1999). Accountability and governance under the new regulatory state. *Australian Journal of Public Administration, 58*(1), 90–97. doi:10.1111/1467-8500.00077

Commission on Global Governance. (1995). *Our global neighbourhood: The report of the Commission on Global Governance*. Oxford University Press.

Considine, M., & Afzal, K. A. (2011). Legitimacy. In M. Bevir, M. (Ed.), The SAGE handbook of governance (369-385). SAGE.

Dalingwater, L. (2017). Shifting governance: TTIP and the public services debate. In J.-B. Velut, L. Dalingwater, V. B. Boullet, & V. Peyronel (Eds.), *Understanding mega-free trade agreements: The political and economic governance of new cross-regionalism* (pp. 86–105). Routledge. doi:10.4324/9781315200989-6

Economic Intelligence Unit. (2016). *Healthcare markets in Europe – What would be the impact of Brexit?* Retrieved March 23, 2018, from https://www.eiu.com/public/topical_report.aspx?campaignid=BrexitHealth

European Commission. (2013, October 10). *Transatlantic trade and investment partnership – solving the regulatory puzzle. Speech by Karel de Gucht.* Retrieved March 23, 2018, from: http:// europa.eu/ rapid/ press- release_ SPEECH- 13- 801_ en.htm

Finkelstein, L. S. (1995). What is global governance? *Global Governance, 1*(3), 367–372. doi:10.1163/19426720-001-03-90000007

Foucault, M. (2007). Security, territory, population: Lectures at the Collège de France 1977– 1978 (M. Senellart, Ed. & G. Burchell, Trans.). Palgrave Macmillan.

Friel, S., Hattersley, L., & Townsend, R. (2014, December 10). Trade policy and public health. *Annual Review of Public Health, 36*(1), 325–344. doi:10.1146/annurev-publhealth-031914-122739 PMID:25494052

Garcia, F. J. (2007). Global justice and the Bretton Woods Institutions. *Journal of International Economic Law, 10*(3), 461–481. doi:10.1093/jiel/jgm022

Hardin, R. (1999). Democracy and collective bads. In I. Shapiro & C. Hacker-Cordón (Eds.), *Democracy's edges* (pp. 63–83). Cambridge University Press. doi:10.1017/CBO9780511586361.006

Hardon, A. P. (2003). New WHO leader should aim for equity and confront undue commercial influences. *Lancet, 361*(9351), 6. doi:10.1016/S0140-6736(03)12177-0 PMID:12521037

Hawkes, N. (2011). 'Irrelevant' WHO outpaced by younger rivals. *BMJ (Clinical Research Ed.), 343*(1), d5012. Retrieved April 6, 2018, from https://www.bmj.com/content/343/bmj.d5012. doi:10.1136/bmj.d5012 PMID:21828204

Healthcare UK. (2016). *Enhancing the NHS through International Engagement*. Crown.

Henderson, J., Dicken, P., Hess, M., Coe, N., & Wai Chung Yeung, H. (2002). Global production networks and the analysis of economic development. *Review of International Political Economy, 9*(3), 436–464. doi:10.1080/09692290210150842

Issenberg, S. (2016). *Outpatients: The astonishing new world of medical tourism*. Global Reports.

Jönsson, C., & Tallberg, J. (Eds.). (2010). *Transnational actors in global governance: Patterns, explanations, and implications*. Palgrave Macmillan. doi:10.1057/9780230283220

Keune, M., Leschke, J., & Watt, A. (Eds.). (2008). *Privatisation and liberalisation of public services in Europe*. Etui.

Koivulsalo, M., Schrecker, T., & Labonté, R. (2009). Globalization and policy space for health and social determinants of health. In R. Labonté, R., T. Schrecker, C. Packer & V. Runnels (Eds.), Globalization and health: Pathways, evidence and policy (pp. 105-130). Routledge.

Korten, D. (2001). *When corporations rule the world* (2nd ed.). Kumarian Press.

Krajewski, M. (2011, November). *Public services in EU trade and investment agreements*. European Federation of Public Service Unions.

Lakhani, N. (2010, January 17). NHS could save millions by flying patients to India. *The Independent*. Retrieved June 2, 2017, from https://www.independent.co.uk/life-style/health-and-families/health-news/nhs-could-save-millions-by-flying-patients-to-india-1870215.html

Lee, K. (2003). *Globalization and health: An introduction*. Palgrave Macmillan. doi:10.1057/9781403943828

Lunt, N., Smith, R., Exworthy, M., Green, S., Horsfall, D., & Mannion, R. (2011). *Medical tourism: treatments, markets and health system implications: A scoping review*. OECD.

MacNaughton, G., & Hunt, P. (2011). A human rights-based approach to social impact assessment. In F. Vanclay & A. M. Esteves (Eds.), *New Directions in Social Impact Assessment: Conceptual and Methodological Advances* (pp. 355–368). Edward Elgar. doi:10.4337/9781781001196.00034

Maier de Kruijff, H., Kainrath, D., & Tannheimer, T. (2016, February). What is the Problem with TTIP? How public services are affected by TTIP and what can be done about it. *FEPS Policy Brief*, 6.

Missoni, N. (2013, January-February). Understanding the impact of global trade liberalization on health systems pursuing universal health coverage. *Value in Health*, *16*(1), S14-S18.

Mitchell, K. (2006). Neoliberal governmentality in the European Union: Education, training and technologies of citizenship. *Environment and Planning: Society and Space*, *24*(2), 389–407. doi:10.1068/d1804

Miyagi, K., Auberson, D., Patel, A. J., & Malata, C. M. (2012, January). The unwritten price of cosmetic tourism: An observational study and cost analysis. *Journal of Plastic, Reconstructive & Aesthetic Surgery; JPRAS*, *65*(1), 22–28. doi:10.1016/j.bjps.2011.07.027 PMID:21865103

OECD. (2004). *Towards high-performing health systems*. OECD.

OECD. (2015). *Health at a glance*. OECD.

Ollila, E., & Koivusalo, M. (2009). Hyvinvointipalvelusta liiketoiminnaksi - terveydenhuollon parantamisen tärkeät valinnat [From welfare services to business opportunities - important choices for healing the healthcare]. In M. Koivusalo, E. Ollila, & A. Alanko (Eds.), *Kansalaisesta kuluttajaksi. Markkinat ja muutos terveydenhuollossa [From citizen to consumer - markets and change in healthcare]* (pp. 21–47). Gaudeamus.

ONS. (2019). *International Passenger Survey*. Retrieved April 4, 2020, from https://www.ons.gov.uk/surveys/informationforhouseholdsandindividuals/householdandindividualsurveys/internationalpassengersurvey

PAHO (Pan American Health Organization), WHO (World Health Organization), & IDRC (International Development Research Centre). (2001). *Research on health sector reforms in Latin America and the Caribbean: Contribution to policymaking*. Paper for pre-summit of the Americas Forum. International Development Research Centre. Retrieved April 7, 2019, from: www.idrc.ca/lacro/docs/conferencias/paho_idrc.html

Peters, B. G. (2011). Institutional theory. In M. Bevir (Ed.), *The SAGE handbook of governance* (pp. 78–90). SAGE. doi:10.4135/9781446200964.n6

Pollard, K. (2019, January 24). The uncertainty in the NHS is pushing more UK patients to consider treatment abroad. *International Medical Travel Journal*. Retrieved March 5, 2020, https://www.imtj.com/blog/brexit-the-ideal-time-to-promote-medical-tourism-to-the-uk-patient/

Public Services International (PSI). (2015, February 3). *Secret proposal for trade in health services in direct conflict with global agenda for health*. Retrieved March 4, 2018, from http://www.world-psi.org/en/secret-proposal-trade-health-services-direct-conflict-global-agenda-health

Putnam, R. (1988). Diplomacy and domestic policies: The logic of two-level games. *International Organization*, *42*(3), 429–460. doi:10.1017/S0020818300027697

Reisman, D. (2014). *Trade in health: Economics, ethics and public policy*. Edward Elgar. doi:10.4337/9781782547211

Rosenau, J. N. (1995). Governance for the Twenty First Century. *Global Governance*, *1*(1), 13–43. doi:10.1163/19426720-001-01-90000004

Scholte, J. A. (2000). *What is "Global" about globalization: A critical introduction*. Palgrave Macmillan.

Skogstad, G. (2005). Contested political authority, risk society, and the transatlantic divide in the regulation of genetic engineering. In E. Grande & L. W. Pauly (Eds.), *Complex Sovereignty: Reconstituting Political Authority in the Twenty-first Century* (pp. 238–260). University of Toronto Press. doi:10.3138/9781442684201-013

Smith, R., Blouin, C., Mirza, Z., Beyer, P., & Drager, N. (2015). *Trade and health: Towards building a national strategy*. WHO Publications.

Thow, A. M., & Gleeson, D. (2017). Advancing public health on the changing global trade and investment agenda: Comment on 'The Trans-Pacific Partnership: Is it everything we feared for health?'. *International Journal of Health Policy and Management*, *6*(5), 295–298. doi:10.15171/ijhpm.2016.129 PMID:28812819

UNCTAD. (2013a). *World Investment Report 2013: Global Value Chains—Investment and Trade for Development*. UNCTAD.

UNCTAD. (2013b). *Non-tariff measures to trade: Economic and policy issues for Developing Countries*. UNCTAD.

Velut, J.-B. (2017). Introduction. In J.-B. Velut, L. Dalingwater, V. Boullet, & V. Peyronel (Eds.), *Understanding mega-free trade agreements: The political and economic governance of new cross-regionalism* (pp. 1–16). Routledge. doi:10.4324/9781315200989-1

Ware, G. (2006). Filling the regulatory gap: The emerging transnational regulator. *Global Governance*, *12*(2), 135–139. doi:10.1163/19426720-01202003

Warrell, H. (2012, August 21). NHS to sell brand worldwide. *Financial Times*. Retrieved April 15, 2020, from https://www.ft.com/content/5765e106-eb19-11e1-984b-00144feab49a

Watt, N. (2014, August 19). Income from private patients soars at NHS hospital trusts. *The Guardian*. Retrieved June 6, 2017, from: https://www.theguardian.com/society/2014/aug/19/private-patient-income-soars-nhs-privatisation

Weiss, M. (2015). *Trading health? Report on the Transatlantic Trade and Investment Partnership*. UK Faculty of Public Health.

WHO/WTO. (2002). *WTO/WHO agreements and public health: A joint study by the WHO and the WTO Secretariat*. WTO/WHO. Retrieved March 3, 2018, from https://www.wto.org/english/tratop_e/serv_e/health_social_e/health_social_e.htm

World Trade Organization (WTO). (2000). *GATS: Scope and definition*. Retrieved April 15, 2020, from https://www.wto.org/english/tratop_e/serv_e/1-scdef_e.htm

World Trade Organization (WTO). (2013). *World Trade Report 2013: Factors shaping the future of world trade*. WTO.

World Trade Organization (WTO). (2014). *Understanding the WTO*. Geneva: WTO. Retrieved April 8, 2018, from https://www.wto.org/english/thewto_e/whatis_e/tif_e/understanding_e.pdf

World Trade Organization (WTO). (2020). *Health and social services*. Retrieved April 15, 2020, from https://www.wto.org/english/tratop_e/serv_e/health_social_e/health_social_e.htm

Zürn, M. (2005). Global governance and legitimacy problems. In D. Held & M. Koenig-Archibugi (Eds.), *Global governance and public accountability* (pp. 136–163). Blackwell.

Conclusion

The National Health Service (NHS) is celebrating its 72nd anniversary this year. The institution still promises to provide services free at the point of use from 'the cradle to the grave', but has experienced a turbulent life since its inception, as we have seen across the various chapters, and particularly since the market reforms of the 1980s. This institution is considered essential as it not only provides health services to the British population but also aims to ensure social cohesion and a strong workforce. Public support of the NHS and maintaining universal access to care remains strong.

Yet such healthcare is also very costly to deliver. British hospitals and public health institutions are currently facing a significant cash crisis, which raises the issue of how long such a funding model can survive. The nature and scope of the work of the NHS has been transformed from ensuring post-war men were fit for work and combating infectious disease to coping with ageing populations and long-term illnesses. Moreover, the reconfiguration of the NHS by successive governments, the changing nature of demand for health and the shifting focus has meant that public healthcare services are no longer considered from a purely 'public good' perspective. Financial pressures, the redefinition of health and social care and globalisation have transformed the public healthcare sector. The current Covid-19 pandemic is also putting unprecedented pressure on health systems across the world and especially those already facing funding pressures such as the NHS.

The key focus of this publication has been the changing dimensions of governance in the NHS and how health workers and stakeholders provide public healthcare services to the nation. However, the various constituents and stakeholders who govern NHS at all multiscalar levels are sometimes seen to be working to different agendas and this tends to cause confusion and conflict, undermining the successful delivery of health services in Britain. The government still continues to play a major role in the running of health services and decision making, even in the new configuration of public health services and the extension of informal networks. Yet this has led to maintaining a top-down approach, reinforced by the managerial dimension and a certain sclerosis in the system. It has also led to what some have called 'the creeping privatisation of the NHS' with ever more emphasis on market-based governance mechanisms reinforced by legislation such as the Health and Social Care Act of 2012. The essential problem with the top-down approach lies with the fact that healthcare reforms have been led by political aspirations rather than public good principles. The increased focus on private sector management practices has somewhat overturned the public service ethos. While such reforms were supposed to make the running of the public health system more efficient, according to a number of country comparisons, the UK is very much middle-of-the-road for health outcomes. The overriding emphasis on targets and the reliance on new providers from the private sector makes for an over complex system. The corrosion of the public good element and the top down approach which prevails is ill-fitted to fulfil the aspirations of the British people to maintain a quality healthcare system, free at the point of use.

Moreover, decentralisation and 'localisation' have only served to fragment the supply of healthcare further. In order for a local approach to function properly, investment must be made in health prevention within local government in parallel with funding given to the national health services. However, additional cuts to budgets have meant that local authorities do not have the means to ensure high standards in health and social care. Within the NHS, a focus on local solutions and further devolution was supposed to represent a move from prescriptive, top-down approaches. Rather than doing away with the top-down approach, further localisation may have served to widen inequities in healthcare supply. The constellation of health workers and stakeholders at a local level make for a very complicated system. As Bevan predicted on the creation of the NHS, devolved power has led to spatial unevenness and poor performance in resource-stretched areas.

To be fair, many localities are trying to establish a joined-up approach towards health and social care provision. The essential problem remains the joining-up of different services. It is very difficult to join-up health and social care and to deal with the expanding needs in long-term care because there is not a single leadership. Short-termism and the rapid turnover and significant departure of staff on the front line also add to the difficulties of acute and primary care providers. Moreover, NHS legislation is vague enough to enable unfair rationalisation and give scope to local administrators, CCGs and the like with severe budget constraints, to use their judgment and, if necessary, unfairly and sometimes illegally ration the supply of healthcare.

There are increasing moves to try to remedy the situation with Integrated Care or Accountable Care Systems. It looks likely in the future that there may be one ring-fenced budget for health and social care to be managed jointly by health and social care providers. A move towards a fully-digitalised or paperless NHS should also support a more integrated and effective system. However, conflicting agendas and a top-down culture, which still permeate the NHS and local administration, will make this a long and complicated process.

Public health service governance has also become more complex as we move increasingly towards a globalised and digitalised health system. Recent health legislation has enabled NHS consultants to engage more in private activity. There would seem to be a real danger of highly qualified staff working in the public sector moving to the private sector and an increase in the number of NHS practitioners offering their talents to a global market. So far, a deficiency of governance in the provision of British global public health services means that there is a significant future risk to adequate provision. A lack of global governance mechanisms to protect health on an international level and failure to take into account the risks to public health of the internationalisation of health services may be highly detrimental to public health services. There also seems to be a tendency for policy makers and joint government initiatives such as Healthcare UK to support NHS bodies in pursuing trade and investment in health services at the expense of other social actors, such as civil society, who rely on policy makers and health organisations to ensure an equitable distribution of health for the population. Thus, the reconfiguration of the public health system in England has made this country even more vulnerable to such risks and opened a new set of governance problems to contend with.

Nevertheless, despite such concerns, the NHS still ensures a universal supply of healthcare, which is considered to be the best way of ensuring even distribution. However, to provide a sustainable health system, often subject to very emotional and emotive reactions, it would seem that a new regulatory regime of health is necessary rather than the current path of further decentralisation, marketisation and internationalisation of public healthcare. The essential problem is that policymakers and analysts in health and trade hold different views, beliefs and have different agendas. When setting policies, defining a clear agenda is not so simple because of the clear imbalance in power in defining policies for global health.

Appendix

LIST OF ABBREVIATIONS

A&E: Accident and Emergency Department
ABPI: Association of the British Pharmaceutical Industry
ACO: Accountable Care Organisation
ACP: Accountable care partnerships
ACS: Accountable care systems
ADASS: Association of Directors of Adult Social Services
BGMA: British Generic Manufacturers Association
BMA: British Medical Association
CAT: Computerised Axial Tomography
CCG: Clinical Commissioning Group
CETA: Comprehensive Economic and Trade Agreement
CHC: Continuing Healthcare
CHP: Community Health Partnership
CQC: Care Quality Commission
COIS: CCG Outcomes Indicator Set
CSDH: Commission on the Social Determinants of Health
CSU: Commissioning Support Unit
DCLG: Department for Communities and Local Government
DHA: District Health Authority
DH/DoH: Department of Health
DfE: Department for Education
DRG: Diagnosis-Related Group
DST: Decision Support Tool
DWP: Department of Work and Pensions
ECB: European Central Bank
EPA: Economic Partnership Agreement
FOI: Freedom of Information

FPH: Faculty of Public Health
FTA: Free Trade Agreement
GATS: General Agreement on Trade in Services
GATT: General Agreement on Tariffs and Trade
GDP: Gross Domestic Product
GP: General Practitioner
GVC: Global Value Chains
HCSA: Health and Social Care Act
HSCIC: Health and Social Care Information Centre
HImPs: Health Improvement Programmes
HLE: Healthy life expectancy
ICS: Investment Court System
IMF: International Monetary Fund
IOM: Institute of Medicines
IRP: Independent Review Panel
ISTC: Independent Sector Treatment Centre
ITC: Independent Treatment Centre
IVF: In Vitro Fertilization
LA: Local Authority
LE: Life Expectancy
LGA: Local Government Association
LHCR: Local Health and Care Records
LIFT: Local Improvement Finance Trust
MCP: Multispecialty Community Provider
MDT: Multidisciplinary Team
MOH: Medical Officer of Health
NAPF: National Performance Assessment Framework
NGO: Non-Governmental Organizations
NHS: National Health Service
NICE: National Institute for Health and Care Excellence
NPfIT: National Programme for IT
NPM: New Public Management
ODI: Overseas Development Institute
OECD: Organiation for Economic Cooperation and Development
ONS: Office for National Statistics
PACS: Primary and Acute Care Systems
PAHO: Pan American Health Organisation
PbR: Payment by Results
PCG: Primary Care Group

PCT: Primary Care Trust
PFI: Private Finance Initiative
PHE: Public Health England
PPI: Patient and Public Involvement
PPP: Public Private Partnership
PPRS: Pharmaceutical Price Regulation Scheme
PRP: Performance-Related Pay
PSA: Public Service Agreement
PTSD: Post-Traumatic Stress Disorder
QALY: Quality-Adjusted Life Year
QIPP: Quality, Innovation Productivity and Prevention
RAF: Royal Air Force
RTA: Regional Trade Agreement
SHA: Strategic Health Authorities
STP: Sustainable and Transformation Plans
TBT: Technical Barriers to Trade
TiSA: Trade in Services Agreement
TNC: Transnational Corporation
TRIPS: Trade Related Aspects of Intellectual Property Rights
TTIP: Transatlantic Trade and Investment Partnership
UKTI: UK Trade and Investment
UNICEF: United Nations International Children's Emergency Fund
WHO: World Health Organisation
WHR: World Health Report

About the Author

Louise Dalingwater is full professor of British politics at Sorbonne Université. She was recruited in September 2019 to further interdisciplinary research between the humanities and medical sciences. Her current research focuses on health policy and healthcare delivery in the United Kingdom, with some comparative research on European health systems (notably France) and global health policy research. Recent publications include a book on the UK service economy, several book chapters on healthcare. She has also authored articles in academic journals including in *Outre Terre* and *The International Journal of Health, Wellness and Society*. She is part of the European Network on Inclusive Approaches to Trade Policymaking (ENIATP) and the Precision Health network (an international research project led by the Universities of Lund and Malmo in Sweden).

Index

P

Q

S

www.ingramcontent.com/pod-product-compliance
Lightning Source LLC
LaVergne TN
LVHW081521300926
849161LV00006B/1252